TABLE OF CONTENTS

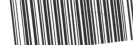

Top 20 Test Taking Tips

1. Carefully follow all the test registration procedures

2. Know the test directions, duration, topics, question types, how many questions

3. Setup a flexible study schedule at least 3-4 weeks before test day

4. Study during the time of day you are most alert, relaxed, and stress free

5. Maximize your learning style; visual learner use visual study aids, auditory learner use auditory study aids

6. Focus on your weakest knowledge base

7. Find a study partner to review with and help clarify questions

8. Practice, practice, practice

9. Get a good night's sleep; don't try to cram the night before the test

10. Eat a well balanced meal

11. Know the exact physical location of the testing site; drive the route to the site prior to test day

12. Bring a set of ear plugs; the testing center could be noisy

13. Wear comfortable, loose fitting, layered clothing to the testing center; prepare for it to be either cold or hot during the test

14. Bring at least 2 current forms of ID to the testing center

15. Arrive to the test early; be prepared to wait and be patient

16. Eliminate the obviously wrong answer choices, then guess the first remaining choice

17. Pace yourself; don't rush, but keep working and move on if you get stuck

18. Maintain a positive attitude even if the test is going poorly

19. Keep your first answer unless you are positive it is wrong

20. Check your work, don't make a careless mistake

Delivery of Care

Healthy People 2020

The first main goal of Healthy People 2020 is to extend life expectancy and to improve a person's quality of life. While life expectancy for Americans has been greatly extended in the last one hundred years, America does not have the highest life expectancy in the world. Also, the life expectancy for different groups within America varies based on gender, race and socio-economic factors. Therefore, the goal of extending life expectancy particularly refers to brining the average age of death into the top three in the world and equalizing life expectancy among all Americans. However, an extended life has very little use if the quality of life is not also improved.

The second goal of Healthy People 2020 is eliminate health inequalities between various groups of people. Women, on average, live longer than men. Some of this difference is due to biological factors, but risk taking and gun use are two other factors that play a role in this disparity. Other areas where differences in health are seen are race, ethnicity, income and educational level.

Nursing boards

The National Council of State Boards of Nursing commissioned a study of the ways in which state boards of nursing approve and accredit schools of nursing. The Practice, Regulation and Education Committee recognized the following five board of nursing methods. First, some boards do not affiliate with national accrediting boards but instead work by themselves. Second, some boards work with national accrediting boards in order to share information. Final approval however comes only from the local board. Third, some boards recognize the national approval as sufficient for accreditation. Next, some boards require that schools first be nationally accredited and then review them for final approval. Finally, some state nursing boards are not involved with the process of approval and accreditation. Instead, the process is done by a separate state government entity.

Data Collection

There are six main ways to collect information during an evaluation. The following outlines how they are used:

1) Questionnaires, surveys, checklists
   - fast method to gather a large amount of data; can be used with any number of people
   - protects participants privacy; not expensive; data doesn't have to be interpreted, making it simple to perform statistical analysis
   - participants not always truthful
   - only tells some information
2) Interviews
   - used to understand in depth information; takes time
   - expensive; generally can not gather large number of samples
3) Documentation review
   - allows information to be gathered on an ongoing process without stopping it- looks at financial records, budgets, emails, etc. - able to view information from start of program
4) Observation
   - enables very accurate information to be learned about the program- real-time data
   - open to interpretation- difficult to analyze statistically
5) Focus groups
   - brings a number of people together to discuss program in depth - participants often candid

- able to gather large amounts of information in a short amount of time
- hard to organize- requires a professional facilitator to conduct properly

6) Case studies
- reviews the experiences of selected individuals
- information gathered can be used for marketing purposes - requires a lot of time
- unable to view a large number of people

Quality and performance principles

The Joint Commission, formerly JCAHO, was created in 1952. The Joint Commission's main focus is accrediting health care institutions, and this is accomplished by measuring institutions against standards like National Patient Safety Goals and Core Measures. The Joint Commission worked with CMS to align Core Measures, which are standards of care that are evidenced-based and backed by research showing that when these standards are performed there are better outcomes for patients. There are currently 14 Core Measurement sets:

• Perinatal Care	• Tobacco Treatment
• Stroke	• Pneumonia Measures
• Venous Thromboembolism	• Immunization
• Heart Failure	• Acute Myocardial Infarction
• Emergency Department	• Children's Asthma Care
• Surgical Care Improvement Project	• Hospital-Based Inpatient Psychiatric Services
• Substance Use	• Hospital Outpatient Department

System theory

Betty Neuman created the systems theory of nursing which concentrates on the patient as a collection of factors all of which must be looked after in order for complete health to occur. There are five factors that must be considered.

1) Physiological - biological processes-traditional focus of health services

2) Psychological - mental processes - environmental stressors

3) Socio-cultural

- Nationality, race, occupation

- education

4) Developmental

- age in years

- maturity level

5) Spiritual

- religious beliefs- values- personal goals

This theory also takes into account the importance of the patient's internal, external and created environments. Finally, there are three types of environmental stressors defined: intrapersonal, problems within the patient; interpersonal, problems between the patient and nearby factors; extra-personal, problems between the patient and long distance factors.

Cultural diversity

Knowledge of **cultural diversity** is important in the field of nursing because the only way a person can be fully understood is by understanding the culture that they come from. Cultural diversity may be defined as differences in race and ethnicity. It is important to recognize the following:

- what the cultural group believes regarding life and death

- the cultural group's definition of fitness and sickness

- the practices the cultural group uses to stay healthy

- beliefs the cultural group has as to what makes people sick
- how the cultural group's healers deal with the sick
- how the nurse's background affects how they care for people

The final point is often overlooked when studying culture's influence on health care services, but until nurses completely understand their own cultural beliefs, it is impossible for them to relate truthfully to others.

Prioritizing patient problems

Once a patient has had a full review and been diagnosed, a nurse should characterize the problems as being of high, intermediate or low priority. High priority problems require emergency treatment or are life threatening in the long term. Intermediate priority problems are those that a nurse can treat but are not life threatening. Low priority problems typify things that can be handled once the patient has left the hospital and are not necessarily medically involved. One way to prioritize non-medical problems is by using Maslow's hierarchy of needs. Maslow's needs, starting with the most basic are: physiological, safety and security, love and belonging, self-esteem and self-actualization. Problems that fit the first and second categories should be dealt with first.

Scheduling methods

There are several methods that can be used for scheduling nurses in health care organizations. Supplemental scheduling, also known as float scheduling, places a number of nurses available to the organization at large so that they can be used when and where they are necessary. For the most part, this type of scheduling has been done away with in favor of using agencies that provide nurses on a daily basis as need arises. Cyclic and block scheduling are similar, with nurses knowing their work time far in advance. Also, both cyclic and block scheduling can be used in conjunction with computerized scheduling. Another factor in scheduling is the number of shifts to place in a 24 hour time period. Health care organizations that do not require around the clock staffing may use two shifts of ten hours each, while those that do require around the clock staffing may use three distinct eight hour shifts, three overlapping ten hour shifts or two twelve hour shifts. There are pluses and minuses to all shift schedules.

Plan of care

Creating a plan of care for patients is an important part of the service process. Written care plans help co-ordinate patient care, decrease the risk of errors and cost, and increase the quality of care. Each hospital or health service organization should use a standard plan of care printed form or format. Often a five-step plan of care is used including the following categories: assessment, problem, goal, treat chosen, how the treatment is working. When taking notes on what treatment is being used, it is important to keep the following questions in mind: 1) What is the treatment? 2) When should each treatment take place? 3) How should the treatment be done? 4) Who should participate in the treatment performance? Some care plans are now inputted solely onto a computer, however if a hand-written plan of care is also done, take time to write neatly and legibly.

Modeling and role-modeling theory

Modeling and Role-Modeling (MRM) theory is a basis for caring for patients as a whole rather than just looking at the illness. Modeling is used in an attempt to find out how the patient sees their environment. Nurses use what they have learned through the modeling process to then help the patient the best they can through role modeling. When working from this theoretical view-point it is very important to gain the patient's trust, build their self-esteem, give them a reason to hope, allow the patient to have as much control as possible, let them know the areas in which they are strong and help them to build on these strengths, and work together to set goals.

Case management

In an effort to lower costs and provide the highest level of care possible, hospitals have begun using case management systems. Third-party payers prefer case management because it allows them to decide if a treatment, hospital stay, medication, etc. was necessary for the patient's health. If the third-party payer believes it was unnecessary then they refuse to pay that portion of the bill. Health care workers appreciate case management because it helps them to co-ordinate patient's care between various disciplines within the system. This co-ordination leads to fewer errors, less time for the patient to remain in the hospital and better continuity of care as the patient moves through the system.

Critical pathways is a type of case management system that was first proposed at the New England Medical Center in Boston in the late 1980's. This system outlines at the beginning of their hospital stay what needs to be done for the patient and when so that their treatment stays on time, proceeds in an orderly fashion and they are discharged on time. A case manager, or head nurse, should be assigned to the patient in order to plan the critical pathway and keep it on track. The nurse is also responsible for explaining the case to other health care providers. This management system lowers the use of resources and costs, but increases the patient's outcome level. A critical path form may include the following information: assessments, consults, procedures, treatments, and activity. It will also list the patient's problems and timeline for care.

Differentiated practice model and PFC

The most common way that nurses are managed is by using the differentiated practice model. This model emphasizes the educational level of the nurses so that within one organization all RN level nurses, for example, have the same amount of responsibility. Another model for nursing practice is known as patient-focused care (PFC). In comparison to the differentiated practice model, PFC is better able to keep costs down and increase health service quality. PFC stresses the use of teams composed of a variety of health professionals. The main resistance to this model is that each team would be self managed and no longer centered around the medical doctor. In order for maximum gain, organizations must first change their philosophy before trying the PFC model.

Physical environment

When planning to build a new facility or renovate an old one, there are several areas of concern. Because health care is now being operated under business models, the patients are one primary concern. It may be advisable to tour other facilities to see what does and does not work. The following six factors are important to have in mind when designing for patients:

- Ease of getting from one area to another.
- Keeping patients from hearing or seeing things that might be upsetting or unpleasant.
- Patient control over whom and what they see and hear while in their room.
- Being sure that the facility is safe and protected.
- Ease of locating special features such as playrooms, cafeterias or gift shops.
- Taking into account the specific needs of different kinds of patients, such as the elderly.

When planning health care facilities it is important that function and design work well together. The basis for judging function comes from state and local laws as well as the HEW Publication 79-14500: Minimum Requirements of Construction and Equipment for Hospitals and Medical Facilities. The following nine factors are also helpful for keeping function appropriate:

- Do not look at the separate areas of the building without looking at how they function as a whole.
- Consider how close some units should be together. For example, the labor and delivery department should be located near the newborn nursery and pediatrics.
- Plan rooms according to the service they will provide.
- Think ahead to the possibility for making the facility larger.
- Keep in mind the ability to change currently defined areas in the future.
- Amount of mechanization desired.
- Separate areas for clean and dirty things.
- Consideration for patient privacy.
- Flow of traffic through the facility.

Redesign

Nurses are on the forefront of changes in the health care field because they work the closest to patients and patients have become the focus of practice. When changing the way a unit works, it is often found that the ineffective practice was being maintained only from habit or tradition. The key word in work redesign is "simplify". If a single person can do a job why ask three people to perform it? Better still is to educate the patients to perform the task themselves, as it will cost far less, and patients who take an interest in their own care get better more quickly than those who are passive. At times, such as when recording medical histories, the patient may even do a better job then someone else would. The four main areas to focus on when redesigning the work of nurses are the types of patients being cared for, resources available, support from management, and the type of nursing being performed.

It is important that nurse administrators be the voice of the nursing staff during building projects, by working on the planning committee. If the building project is large and will take years to accomplish, then a full time nurse advisor should be assigned to the project. There are six important things that the nurse advisor should be sure to work on:

- Be sure that the nursing unit is involved with the planning and design development.
- Find information and reference sources.
- Study new ideas in architecture, medical treatment facilities and technological advances.
- Look over organization ideas and outline the necessary appliances and space for the nursing staff.
- Work to explain medical terminology and concepts to the project designer, architect, building code enforcers, etc.
- Keep watch over the project as it is built to make sure it follows all pre-arranged ideas.

Interior design

In the past, the hospital environment was cold and sterile and little thought above functionality was put into their interior design. However, there are now magazines devoted to the interior design of hospitals and health care facilities and professionals who specialize in making the environment more patient-friendly. Some examples that can be used to guide plans for interior design follow:

- use art work which is culturally familiar to patient groups
- use colors to create a cheerful, soothing or relaxed atmosphere
- use as much natural light as possible
- windows in every patient room
- using repeating textures or colors to identify particular units
- make patient rooms as home-like as possible
- have public areas be as open and light as possible
- create interior courtyard gardens for patients who are unable to leave the grounds
- use comfortable seating in waiting rooms

Performance improvement

Performance improvement (PI) looks at how individuals are working and how they might work better. There are ten important factors that are fundamental to PI:

1) Concentrate on end results.
2) Look at how the entire organization plays a role in each individual's work.
3) Create services that are more adequate for the patient.
4) Help individuals work together and form teams.
5) Look at what the individual is doing in comparison to what the organization needs.
6) Look at why an individual is working in a specific way.
7) Carefully create changes to maximize outcome potential.
8) Use innovation to come up with new ways to work.
9) Carefully execute the changes.
10) Attentively look at what happens as a result of the changes made.

Report cards

Report cards, also known as scorecards, are used to assess how well a program or organization has been functioning and how well it may be able to function in the future. Report cards measure many different aspects in order to attempt to present the whole picture. Some of these measurements include income, customer satisfaction, staff satisfaction and growth. They also help to identify the factors that are influencing the program. These factors are broken down into four separate categories. First are environmental factors, the things outside of the organization's control. Second are organizational factors, the internal workings of the organization. Next are the departmental factors, the unit levels' cause and effects. Finally, there are the individual factors, the ways in which programs are managed and how leaders function.

Continuous quality improvement

Continuous quality improvement (CQI) is a strategy for making changes to a program very often without interrupting the program's work. In CQI, importance is placed on how things are being done and data analysis is used to make changes. Success is based on whether or not a patient's needs are met. Quality is based on what the patient expects. There are seven basic steps in CQI:

1) Create a group that understands the program.
2) Create clearly defined goals.
3) Learn what patients' needs are.
4) Decide on a way to measure whether the program is working to its full potential.
5) Think of ways that might make the program better.
6) Conduct research and analyze data to make the best decision possible.
7) Test the changes and reanalyze.

Access to care

Access to care has become an increasing problem in America. In 2005, there were several positive improvements in access and many negative factors in access. Many health care organizations have finally begun to spend money to make their facilities larger in order to raise the number of patients that they can see. This is especially true of emergency rooms. Many private doctor's offices are beginning to have equipment on site that just a few years ago was found only in hospitals, including ultrasound machines and positron emission tomography (PET) scanners. While these two factors have improved access to care for some people, such as those in rural areas, they have also made services more expensive and therefore more difficult to access by people without insurance. To continue with financial matters, the fact that health service organizations have begun to market themselves as businesses has increased competition and lowered prices in some areas.

Unfortunately, there are still no real strategies for controlling the ever increasing cost of health care.

Americans with Disabilities Act

The Americans with Disabilities Act (ADA) "prevents discrimination on the basis of disability" in six main areas. The ADA defines a disability as "a person who has a physical or mental impairment that substantially limits one or more major life activities." The ADA does not list specific disabilities that are covered under its regulations. Title I of the ADA states that people with disabilities cannot be discriminated against in the workplace. An employer must make an effort to help the employee with a disability perform well on the job and may not punish them with lower pay, withholding promotions, etc.

Title II of the ADA states that all state and local governments make all of their programs available to people with disabilities. These programs include public transportation, parks and recreation, health care and public education. Governments must also take into account people with disabilities when designing public buildings, and modify existing buildings or change venues when they are inaccessible to people with disabilities. Title III of the ADA requires that all privately owned publicly accessible facilities and transportation must accommodate people with disabilities. Facilities may be defined as hospitals and other health care providers, restaurants, hotels, retail stores and private schools. Transportation refers to privately owned companies that own and or operate buses, trains, planes, etc. All factories, warehouses and other commercial facilities must use the ADA's architectural guide when altering existing buildings or constructing new ones.

The Federal Communication Commission (FCC) has set standards in regards to Title IV of the ADA. This portion refers to the use of telephones by people who have hearing and speech disabilities. Telecommunications relay services that allow for the use of telecommunications devices for the deaf, also known as teletypewriters, must be available to and easily accessible for people with disabilities. This pertains to public phone booths, cell phones, and operator services, for example, and is overseen by the FCC. In 1988 the Fair Housing Act was enacted to protect people from housing discrimination on the basis of disability as well as other factors. Owners or managers of housing facilities must make reasonable accommodations in order to allow people with disabilities to live on their property. For example, someone who is blind and uses a guide dog may be able to reside in an apartment despite a no pet policy.

Crisis management

There are several situations in which crisis management might be used, such as in the event of a power outage or something more long term such as a cash flow problem. Each organization should have a crisis management plan on file and all employees should be routinely briefed on its particulars. There are five steps that should be a part of the crisis management scheme.
- determine why the crisis is happening
- decide if the reasons for the crisis will have long term effects or only short term effects on the organization
- determine what is most likely to happen as events unfold
- focus on the individuals who can help the most and get them working on the most fundamental problems first
- look for ways to learn or grow from the crisis event

Occupational Safety and Health Act

In 1991 the Occupational Safety and Health Act (OSHA) was established in an attempt to protect employees from harm in the workplace. All health care agencies must include OSHA guidelines in their own safety practice procedures and should have a designated OSHA administrator to oversee compliance to the OSHA regulations. There are five main areas in which OSHA guidelines are involved: exposure control, universal precautions, housekeeping, high-risk exposure and training. For each area, the health care agency must have a specific plan in place, keep workers informed of updates or changes, and post reminders in prominent places. Items necessary for the implementation guidelines must be provided to employees free of charge and kept in easily accessible areas. In order to minimize risk, health care workers should be given immunizations and screened for possible exposure on a regular basis. Training on OSHA practices and procedures should be compulsory rather than voluntary.

Strategic planning

Strategic planning is the process by which administrators make high-risk decisions using all available information on how the decision will effect the organization. There are six steps for proper strategic planning:
1) Decide how the decision making process will occur.
2) Come up with a mission statement or look over the current mission statement in order to stay focused on long-term organizational goals.
3) Look over the external factors involved in the process.
4) Analyze the internal factors involved in the process.
5) State what will be achieved.
6) Come up with a number of valid possible decisions that meet all stated criteria.

The first step in evaluating external factors during the strategic planning process is to examine the economy. In today's environment, all levels of the economy should be looked at including international, national, state and local because all play a role in the financing of health care. Political factors on both a national and local level must also be taken under consideration. National politics play a role in the funding for and availability of sex education, family planning and birth control. Local politics influence who has access to care. Another critical issue in strategic planning is market trends. For example, in the last ten years more people have been turning to non-traditional medical services such as acupuncture and herbal remedies, which in turn have influenced some insurance companies and their reimbursement of such treatments as well as mainstream hospitals hiring and advertising specialists in non-traditional medicine.

Trends in technology is another factor that must be carefully considered when making strategic planning assessments. Now healthcare professionals must not only stay on top of the latest medical advancements such as in the field of biotechnology but in the ever increasingly complex computer systems used in the administrative field. The population of America is growing older and with this development an increased pressure on geriatric services. Other social factors that come into play when forecasting long-range outcomes are the early return to work faced by new mothers, single parent households, and gay and lesbian cohabitation.

Several governmental agencies must be watched for proposed and scheduled changes to their regulatory rules. These agencies include the Occupational Safety and Health Administration as well as local health and state service agencies. In order to fully understand the organization's standing within the community, several factors can be compared between one health service facility and another. Factors such as occupancy rates, medical specialists, and types of patients seen can help the planner place the importance of their facility within the community. Financial factors also play a role in facility comparison. It is also important to determine how the community, patients, doctors and nurses feel about the organization. Finally, issues in manpower are especially important to strategic planning. The predicted number of nurses, general practitioners, and specialists can help the administrator to plan for starting or increasing some services while decreasing or ending others.

Step four in the strategic planning continuum is conducting an internal assessment. Where the organization is particularly strong or areas that need improvement should be highlighted. Learning how the members of an organization communicate is also important if any plan is to work successfully. The following list summarizes the reaming factors important to internal assessment:

- management structure and style
- staff statistics in areas such as education, experience and age
- budget
- advertising and educational outreach programs
- services offered
- organizational structure and culture
- the buildings and infrastructure
- computer resources
- leadership structure and style

The fifth step for administrators working with the strategic framework is goal setting. Goals should be attainable and described in fullest detail. Next, possible solutions should be created using brain storming, Delphi activities, roundtable discussions, etc. Possible solutions can be described as practical, ready for immediate application; incremental, available over time after pursuing specific steps; and radical, those solutions that would mean changing in large ways. In the final steps of strategic planning solutions are chosen, developed and put into place. Once in place, the plan should be evaluated using the critical path method or the program evaluation review technique. Following evaluations, adjustments can be made in order to make the new program run at top performance.

Program planning management

There are six factors that should be in place in order to effect positive program planning management:

1) Start with the mission statement and work outwards, forming goals and then programs that work together.

2) Make use of strategic planning methods to increase the fit of the plan to the organization's overall philosophy.

3) If the organization is a corporation, be sure to have board members involved in the planning process.

4) Remember that program planning is a team effort, not the task of a lone individual.

5) Receive feedback from current and potential customers throughout the planning process to be sure that the plan is viable.

6) No plan will be perfect; some things will need to be adjusted.

Mission statement

Organizations let people know why they are in business by declaring a formal mission statement. An example of a mission statement for a public hospital might be, "Washington County Hospital will serve the citizens of our area by maintaining a high quality of health care and outreach programs." A mission statement not only lets the public understand the function of an organization but also guides the administrative staff in their pursuit of a structure to plan the management style. It is important for all of the parties with an interest in the organization to decide together what the mission statement should outline and what it means exactly. From time to time the functioning of the organization should be reviewed to be sure that it is living up to its mission statement. If the organization is failing in its stated goals then either the management must change its ways or the mission statement must be revised.

Goals

There are two general types of goals: short-term and long-term. Typically, short-term goals take a week or less to accomplish. Short-term goals are very important when working with clients because hospital stays last on average two to three days. These goals usually focus on getting better. Long-term goals may take months to accomplish although it is important to set a time limits to strengthen motivation. These goals usually focus on staying better. When working with patients it is important to keep client-centered goals in mind. Patients and nurses work together to create health goals. Because the patient plays such a large role in creating the goals, they often feel more invested in completing them. If a patient is not able to make goals for themselves then the nurses should work with guardians, family member or other health practitioners to form goals for them.

Goals based vs. process based evaluations

When programs have been created to achieve specific goals, the goals based evaluation model can be helpful for deciding if the goals have been met properly. The following factors should be taken into account during the evaluation:

- The way in which goals were determined
- At what point on the agenda the program is currently
- List resources that are needed and/or unavailable
- Think about making changes in order to keep program on task

Process based evaluations focus on how the program is working. There are several factors that need to be addressed when completing a process based evaluation:

- How are decisions regarding production made?
- Discover how the employees are delivering the service. What are the current marketing strategies?
- Check customer satisfaction.
- Check employee satisfaction.
- Ask for customer and employee ideas for making the program better.
- Learn what customers and employees are complaining about.

Contingency planning

Contingency plans are made in the event of catastrophic events such as natural disasters. A group of individuals representing each area of the health care organization should meet to develop contingency plans so that nothing is overlooked. First, a list of all possible events should be developed and then ranked based on likelihood and amount of impact they might have. Next, a plan should be developed for each catastrophic event, which details what to do immediately following the event and what should be done to bring the organization back up to full function. Once staff have been briefed on a plan, a drill should take place to test the plan's effectiveness. Afterward, opinions from the staff should be taken into account for modifying the existing plan. Finally, contingency plans should be kept up to date with staff receiving refresher courses and drills at regular intervals.

Marketing

Marketing in health care is used to learn what consumers need and how to fulfill those needs in a cost effective manner. Surveys, whether done by the organization itself or from viewing information from other surveys, can help to determine these needs. Market share is defined as the amount of a particular service that one health care organization has in comparison to other organizations in the area. Market penetration is defined by how well known the organization has made its name and brand of services to potential customers. Two cost effective ways to advertise are by creating an organizational web site on the Internet and to feed the media public interest stories that tell the public what a caring institution the organization is.

Image building

It is important for an organization to form a mission statement and from this decide on the image they wish to project upon the public. This image should be understood by all staff members. Staff members should also be taught how to spread the image. Nurses are especially important in providing a positive image in advertising, and because of the nursing shortage nurses have the opportunity to teach people about the wide variety of jobs they do in order to bring new nurses to the profession. Large organizations generally hire a public relations manager to act as an official speaker for the organization. The public relations manager deals with the media, police, workers and consumers. It is their job to make sure the organization's message stays the same and to keep problems under control.

Community assessment

There are ten steps that must be completed when undertaking a health assessment of the community:
1) Form an assessment group.
   - Choose qualified hardworking individuals. - Explain in detail what will be expected. - Create a framework for leadership.
2) Decide what is needed to complete the assessment and obtain it.
   - Create a budget. - Find resources already at hand.
   - Make a backup plan.

3) Find and speak with members of the community that are willing to help.
   - Decide the boundaries of the community. - Give important duties to community volunteers.
   - Settle on how communications will take place.
4) Assemble, evaluate and state information found.
   - Primary data: information gathered by the team.
   - Secondary data: information already available.
5) Decide what is important.
   - Have team member submit ideas. - Allow the team to vote on final decisions.
6) Expand the underlying information.
   - Think of what may be causing the problems found. -Gather more information. - Focus on small things first.
7) Determine goals.
   - Be "SMART": Specific, Measurable, Attainable, Resources, Time limits.
8) Decide how goals will be achieved.
   - Look to see what other groups have done in similar situations; stay acquainted with research in the area of importance; figure out how to make evaluations.
9) Write the final report.
   - List team members, sources of funds, community volunteers and other human resources used.
   - Briefly outline the reasons for conducting the assessment. - Present information found.
10) Keep the process going.
   - Look over what the team needs to do next. Change the plan if necessary.
   - Continue to sample information from the community.

Decision making

Prescriptive model

Ethical decisions may be reached by using the prescriptive model of decision making. This model urges the decision maker(s) to be rational and to strive for the absolute best possible outcome. There are four steps that the decision maker(s) must move through and that aid the process. First, the problem must be defined and studied. Second, all rational solutions to the problem should be listed. Next, each solution is looked at in depth, identifying any negative or positive consequences that could arise as the result of choosing that particular solution. Finally, the solution that will bring about the best outcome is chosen.

Descriptive model

In contrast to the time intensive prescriptive model, the descriptive model of decision making understands that health care professionals must often make quick decision without looking at every possible solution. Instead of coming to the optimal solution the descriptive model only requires that the solution be "satisficing" or acceptable. This model has five steps that the decision maker must move through and that aid the process. First, the problem must be defined and studied. Second, what conditions must be met in order for a solution to be acceptable must be decided upon. Third, various solutions should be listed. Next, each possible solution is looked at to see if it would create a satisfising outcome. Finally, the acceptable solution is chosen.

Applied ethics

Applied ethics use philosophical ideas to develop solutions for problems that actually occur. One method used in applied ethics is casuistry, also known as case-based reasoning. Casuistry compares historical examples of ethical problems with the current ethical problem in order to come to a solution that will be in the best interest of all involved parties. The biggest problem with casuistry is in finding the relevant historical case to use as a comparison. Two opposing methods used in applied ethics are utilitarianism and deontology. The utilitarian method states that the correct solution is the one that results in the most good no matter how the solution is brought about. On the other hand, the deontological method states that the solution is not as important as the way in which the solution is reached.

Feasibility studies

Feasibility studies are conducted before a project is undertaken to see if the project will be successful or not. They can also be used to determine which of several possible solutions would best fix a specific problem. There are six factors:

1) Financial - is the solution within the organization's budget -will the solution be profitable
2) Technical - is it mechanically possible to construct the solution - will the project be hard to construct
3) Itinerary - Is there enough time to complete the project - will creating the solution interrupt the organization too much
4) Organizational - Will the company be willing to support the decision. Will it be too upsetting for the company
5) Cultural - how will the project effect the local community
6) Legal - is the solution completely legal - will there be any challenges to the decision in court

Informatics

Nursing informatics, also known as information science, is the process of combining health care models with theories from information management. The research being done in this area continues to improve patients' quality of care, while making the work for nurses less complicated and more efficient. Informatics allows the nurse administrator to manage data and to use the data to solve problems within the unit. The American Nursing Association has decided that one system of this type should be adopted by all nursing programs in order to allow different organizations to share information and to be sure that all nurses receive the same educational standards in computer science and information technology. The ANA stresses that the following points are most important for creating a nationwide structure:

- classification: how items are grouped together
- database: how files are grouped together
- dataset: information that is similar
- data element: small meaningful bits of information
- language: computer code
- nomenclature and vocabulary: how items are named
- taxonomy: how vocabulary is grouped together

Legal, Regulatory, and Ethical Issues

Medicare

Medicare is government supported insurance available to individuals over age 65, in end-stage renal disease, or those under 65 with specified disabilities. There are two parts of Medicare: part A, hospitalization insurance for short term emergency care; part B, for doctor visits and outpatient services. Some services are paid according to a flat rate with the rest being paid for out of pocket by the client or by the client's supplemental insurance plan. Other services are reimbursed according to a percentage chart such as 80% Medicare and 20% client. Under certain diagnosis, the practitioner must accept the Medicare benefit as payment in full without trying to bill the client. Exact payment by the government is calculated by the DRG classification system. Services not covered by Medicare include long-term care, preventative health measures, eye exams and glasses, hearing exams and hearing aids, and dental care, unless care is needed in an emergency situation.

Resource Utilization Groups

Resource Utilization Groups (RUG-III) is a system under Medicare PPS that makes payments based on what resources within a long-term care facility should be used according to the patient's diagnosis. There are 44 RUG-III groups each of which state a specific reimbursement amount. Payments vary within each group according to the facility's location. Money is given for time spent with a health care practitioner, medications, food, laundry, and facilities for example. The patient's RUG-III is determined by the minimum data set (MDS). The MDS is a standardized assessment instrument used by nurses to gather information on the patient's statues including their activities of daily living (ADLs), mental status, and medical needs. The MDS and therefore, RUG-III may change over the course of a patient's stay and is assessed on the 5th, 14th, 30th, 60th, and 90th days following admission or days following the start of Medicare Part A payment eligibility.

Home Health Resource Groups

Home Health Resource Groups (HHRG) is a classification system used by Medicare as part of its prospective payment system for providers of in-home health care services. There are 80 groups into which a patient may be classified. The classification into an HHRG is determined by the Outcome and Assessment Information Set (OASIS). OASIS covers such categories as physical and mental assessments, how the family is working, the home environment, what the patient is able to do for themselves and what they need help with. Nursing in the home setting may be provided for such problems as an inability to practice self-care or for hygiene due to pain, high risk for infection due to acquired immunity deficiency, and the inability to ingest food due to throat impairment.

Medicaid

Medicaid is a state regulated government sponsored health insurance for people living well below the poverty line. Medicaid is used in large part to pay for health services for pregnant women, infants and young children. During the 1980's Medicaid funding was drastically cut which led in to huge increases in infant mortality rates. Physicians and hospitals are paid only a flat fee for providing care to Medicaid patients and are not reimbursed the remaining amount and so try to limit the amount of Medicaid patients seen. Unlike Medicare, which is an entitlement program, Medicaid is a social welfare program, which relies on both state and federal funds. Medicaid was created through Title XIX of the Social Security Act on July 30, 1965.

Health Maintenance Organizations

Health Maintenance Organizations (HMOs) were created in 1973 to try to lower health costs by encouraging competition among providers to charge lower prices in order to become part of the HMO system. People who are enrolled in an HMO pay premiums to the HMO who in turn pays the health care provider. The HMOs focus on providing preventative health care in order to help keep costs down. Other ways in which costs are controlled include limiting services depending on a diagnosis, the use of second opinions and pre-approval by the HMO before certain services are rendered.

There are four types of HMOs. An independent practice association HMO contracts health care services through privately practicing doctors. Sometimes HMOs may group their contracted physicians into a single building or complex, which is known as group practice. Rather than contracting private practicing doctors, staff model HMOs hire physicians directly to work at specific locations. Finally, HMOs may also contract medical groups to service clients in particular areas.

Preferred Provider Organizations

Preferred Provider Organizations (PPOs) also known as industry-based health plans are a type of managed care system. Private insurance companies or large corporations may bargain with groups of physicians or other health care providers to provide health care to their participants at specified low rates. Generally individuals can choose to use providers outside of their PPO however when they use the health care providers listed through their PPO they save considerable amounts of money. For all but basic wellness check-ups and preventative medical interventions clients must have pre-approval from the PPO or be referred from a participating PPO doctor. While health care providers may make less money per individual, they benefit overall by having a large client pool and receiving fast assured payments.

Capitated systems

The capitated system is a relatively new type of payment scheme that places financial risks onto the health care provider. Insurance companies or large corporations pay the service provider according to the number of people covered under the policy rather than paying for the actual services. Providers who enter into capitated delivery systems must keep strict control over their budget because no more funds will come available once the arranged fee is paid. The delivery focus in capitated systems is preventative health care and keeping people at a manageable level of health because these services are far less expensive than treating illness. There is also a tendency to use expensive assessment measures. Research has not shown that patient care suffers from these differences.

Methods of repayment

Per diem, literally "by the day", is a third party repayment plan mostly used by Health Maintenance Organizations (HMOs). The HMO pays the hospital a pre-determined amount of money for each day the patient is in the hospital regardless of what the hospital does for the patient. The payment amount may be based on the patient's ward within the hospital or may be the same no matter what ward the patient is on. If the HMO decides that it was unnecessary for the patient to have been hospitalized on certain days it will refuse payment for those days. Indemnity plans, also known as fee-for-service, cover a set percentage of the medical bill. In the past these plan paid the same set percentage regardless of the total cost. However, some have moved to a case management strategy in an effort to lower cost.

Diagnostic related groups

Diagnostic related groups (DRGs) are used to calculate prospective repayment within the health care field. The theory of DRGs is that if only a set amount of money is paid out for specific treatment procedures then the health care facility will find a way to lower costs in order to realize a profit from the set amount. In reality however this systems of DRGs can lead to a reduction in the quality of care patients receive because the facility will only care for the individual according to the DRG repayment guideline. Currently there are 492 DRGs within Medicare Part A. Examples of DRGs include newborn, heart failure and pneumonia.

Health Insurance Portability and Accountability Act

The Health Insurance Portability and Accountability Act (HIPAA) gives many guaranteed rights to individuals regarding health insurance. HIPAA puts limitations on which pre-existing medical conditions insurance companies can exclude from coverage. According to HIPAA it is the individual states' right to regulate the health insurance business. HIPAA does not allow people to be excluded from coverage or be charged more because of their health status. Title II of HIPAA known as the Administrative Simplification Provisions forced the Department of Health and Human Services to create a nationwide standard for sending information electronically and for keeping computerized records safe from unauthorized viewers. It is hoped that HIPAA will lead to universal health coverage in the United States and that Title II of HIPAA will allow any health facility to access a patient's information quickly and easily.

Nuremberg Code

The Nuremberg Code developed during the trial of Nazi doctors is the basis for the Code of Federal Regulation Title 45 Volume 46 published by the United States

Department of Health and Human Services, which administrates research that is done with federal funding. The Code has ten points. 1) Any person used in research must give their permission after being told about the experiment. 2) The research must be important and helpful in nature. 3) Research should first be tried on animals. 4) If at all possible, the subjects should not have any pain because of the research. 5) If it is thought that death will occur because of the research then the study should not be done. 6) The potential benefits should outweigh any potential risks associated with the study. 7) The investigators must take all necessary precautions to avoid injury to the subjects. 8) Investigators should be educated in the field of study they are researching. 9) Subjects must be allowed to leave the study at any time. 10) Investigators should stop the study if they are worried that harm may befall the subjects.

Patient Self Determination Act

The Patient Self Determination Act was part of the Omnibus Budget Reconciliation Act of 1990 and is required to be followed by all health care agencies that receive Medicaid funding. This act states that all people have the right to refuse medical care and should be given a written statement that fully explains their rights as patients. If a person is unable to make medical decisions for themselves due to being a minor, mentally incompetent or otherwise impaired then a legal guardian should sign on their behalf. The important part of this act is that the decision be "informed" meaning that the patient or guardian understand fully the risks and benefits attached to any procedure.

Another factor of this act deals with **advanced medical directives**. There are two types of advanced medical directives: living will and health proxies. An individual creates a living will which states what treatments they choose to accept or deny in the event that they are in some way impaired and terminally ill. Health proxies are people appointed to make medical decisions for an individual in case of impairment.

Medical malpractice

Medical malpractice is defined as negligence on the part of a health care provider that causes a patient to be injured. In order to prove negligence the plaintiff, the patient or someone speaking for them, must demonstrate that the following four things are true. First, they must show that the defendant, the health care provider or hospital, had a legal duty to take care of them. Second, they must prove that the defendant acted outside the "standard of care". Next, they must establish that the action of the defendant was the event that caused the injury. Finally, they must demonstrate that damages occurred. Damages may be either a loss of money or mental anguish brought about by the injury. Expert witnesses, someone whom the Court believes is qualified in the area under scrutiny, may be called by either plaintiff or defendant in an effort to win the case.

Lawsuits regarding medical malpractice have been highly publicized over the last fifteen years leading many people to believe that the vast majority is frivolous and that high monetary rewards are the reason medical malpractice insurance is so expensive. In a study performed by David M. Studdert, et al. the exact opposite was found to be true. From a sample of 1452 closed malpractice claims 80% involved extreme disabilities or death. Of the remaining 20%: 3% showed no detrimental outcome, 4% claimed psychological or emotional injury, and less than 1% dealt with informed consent problems. A full 54% of money paid to the injured parties was for the litigation costs. The vast majority of litigation expenses, 80%, were paid in cases where the injury was due to harmful error on the part of the health care practitioner. Showing that it is administrative costs and valid lawsuits are the true reasons for the increase in insurance costs.

Negligence is defined as the injury to a person due to a breach in standard of care. There are three laws by which an employer can be sued because of the negligent actions of their employees: negligent hiring, negligent entrustment, and vicarious liability. If an employer hires an individual with the knowledge that the individual has a history of negligence then the employer can be charged with negligent hiring if the individual is accused of negligence in the new job. Negligent hiring is typically used in cases involving a misuse of authority. On the other hand, negligent entrustment generally involves physical injury. Negligent entrustment occurs when an employer assigns a duty to an employee for which the employee is not qualified for or sufficiently trained. Finally, even if the employer did not act negligently they still may be sued for negligence under the "agency theory."

Lawsuits

There are many reasons why a nurse can be sued for malpractice. The following reasons can be used if the nurse actually makes a mistake or if someone thinks they did. In addition, the nurse can be sued if a junior nurse under their supervision commits an error. If the nurse is not the original target of the lawsuit, the primary defendant may sue the nurse. Some reasons lawsuits are filed include:

- oversight made during patient monitoring
- inaccuracy created in the patient's files regarding medical procedures or treatments
- a physician believes the nurse did not follow instructions
- lack of full patient consent due to patient not receiving adequate information
- helping anyone with a medical problem while not at work

Health Care Fraud and Abuse Control Program

The Health Care Fraud and Abuse Control Program (HCFAC) was created in 1996 by the Department of Health and Human Services to prevent fraud, waste, and abuse in the Medicaid and Medicare systems. HCPAC is administered by the Office of Inspector General (OIG). Not only does the HCFAC work to prevent problems but also enforces rules and collects money improperly appropriated. The HCFAC has five main goals:

1) to organize all levels of law enforcement attempts to crack down on the problem of fraud, waste, and abuse
2) to administer examinations, financial checks, and assessments concerning government payments for Medicaid and Medicare bills
3) to help implement countermeasures against deception
4) to tell the health care industry exactly what practices are wrong
5) to create a nationwide computerized network detailing the judgments against deceitful providers

There are several areas where Medicare and Medicaid fraud are most likely to occur. Common fraud cases in nursing homes include labeling normal patients as hospice patients, ordering supplies for one patient then using them with other patients, and billing for mental health services that were not necessary. Common fraud cases in home health care services include charging too much for oxygen tanks and feeding supplies and prescribing too much medication. Another place in which fraud and abuse of the system are widespread is in the durable medical equipment (DME) area. The pricing structure set up by congress in 1987 is prone to misuse, but obtaining a license to sell DME has become much more difficult due to a crackdown on fraudulent businesses. Finally, some companies who sell secondary coverage sometimes use unethical marketing practices to lure individuals to pay for things they do not need which puts them under scrutiny from the federal government.

Standards for patient care

The American Nursing Association (ANA) outlines patient care standards in five general areas.

1) Assessment- Nurse gets information from client about their health. - Information gather continues throughout the patient's stay. - Assessment follows an exact plan. - Health history may be gotten from other health care professionals or family members.

2) Diagnosis - Nurse looks over information gathered for deciding what is wrong with the patient. - Diagnosis is documented in care plan. - Consults with others as needed. - Nurse outlines future outcomes. - Uses outcomes to create goals. - Outcomes are pragmatic. - Outcomes are given with a schedule.

3) Planning - Nurse creates care plan outlining treatments and predicted outcomes. - Plan of care specific to each client. - Plan is kept up to date.- Plan is written out.

4) Implementation - Nurse begins treatment. - Treatment based on plan of care. - Treatment is safe and ethical. - Treatment is written down.

5) Evaluation- Nurse checks to see if patient is reaching goals. - Evaluation is constant and follows and exact plan. - How the patient responds to each treatment is recorded.

The American Nursing Association (ANA) lists a number of standards for professional performance. The responsibilities of a nurse include:

- reviewing how good the practice in an organization is and how much the practice is helping the patient
- making sure they are following all rules and policies concerning their work
- keeping up with nursing information through continuing education
- helping other nurses to grow in their field
- making decisions and treat patients ethically

- working with their patients and other health care workers to give the patients the best possible care
- keeping up with the latest research and apply findings to their work
- thinking about safety, how well something works and how much it will cost when creating plans of care and when treating patients.

Protocols and standing orders

A protocol is a formal set of regulations used when diagnosing or treating patients. General protocols may be created for the entire health care organization such as directions for calling codes or dealing with safety threats. Protocols created at the until level are usually more specific and might be about how often a patient's blood pressure should be taken and noted or what questions should be asked when taking a patient's medical history. Standing orders are similar to protocols as they are also formal written instructions. However, standing orders are specific to each patient. Generally the nurse and physician will work together to create standing orders. Standing orders may also be put in place by the doctor in case she is unobtainable when the patient needs something. These orders may specify the amount and type of pain medication allowed or what to do if the patient's temperature gets very high.

Privacy and confidentiality

Privacy and **confidentiality** are two words often associated with medical ethics. Privacy for the patients in the physical sense refers to the idea that only necessary health professionals are allowed to view the patient and in the auditory sense that no one should be able to overhear conversations regarding patients. Confidentiality deals with patient information. Only those medical professionals directly assigned to a case should have full access to a patient's file. When consulting with other health professionals the nurse should provide only the information necessary for help and such identifying facts as patient name should be kept private. Strict protocols should be in place regarding the sharing of patient information with outside parties like insurance companies. However, confidentiality between nurse and patient is not absolute. The nurse may alert police or others if the patient is a threat.

Ethics

The American Heritage Dictionary defines ethics as "that branch of philosophy dealing with values relating to human conduct, with respect to the rightness and wrongness of certain actions and to the goodness and badness of the motives and ends of such actions." Health care ethics address medical issues, the distribution of limited resources, experiments involving people, and health legislature. Health care ethics attempts to give individuals a way to decide what is best for a patient when there is a conflict concerning moral questions. One ethical conflict that is constantly debated is the definition of death. It is possible to keep a person, who has no brain waves and the inability to breath on their own, alive via medical technology for a very long time. It is possible but is it ethical? There are a number of factors to take into consideration of any ethical medical question besides the personal belief of the individuals involved. They must also consider appropriate use of resources, the patient's wishes, and medical diagnosis.

Code of Ethics for Nurses with Interpretive Statements
Code of Ethics for Nurses with Interpretive Statements was first begun in 1995 and written by the American Nursing Association Board of Directors and the Congress on Nursing Practice in joint cooperation. The Code currently consists of nine provisions.

The first provision states that it is the nurse's responsibility to treat each patient the same with kindness and consideration. This deals with the treatment of patients in an ethical manner. There are four subdivisions of this first provision:

1) Respect for human dignity
   - all people have the same fundamental rights
   - nurses must look after each persons individual needs
2) Relationship to patients
   - all people have a right to health care
   - nurses do not judge individuals
   - nurses give courtesy to all people
3) The nature of health problems
   - human rights are not diminished because of medical diagnosis
   - nurses should try to make their patients as comfortable as possible
   - nurses should provide death with dignity
   - nurses must not give medication only to bring death
4) The right to self-determination
   - the rights of individuals also pertain to people who the nurse works with
   - nurses must not act in any way prejudiced

The second provision says that the paramount duty of the nurse is to the patient no matter how "patient" is defined. This provision also has four subdivisions:

1) Primacy of the patient's interests- plans of care must be made in a way that is unique to each individual patient. Nurses work to help solve problems between patients and family members
2) Conflict of interest for nurses - when problems arise between the patient's needs and the needs or wants of the health care organization the nurse works to keep the patient's needs paramount

3) Collaboration- collaboration is people working together to solve problems. - nurses should work to keep collaboration working in their organization - clinical nurses must work with administrative nurses for the good patients

4) Professional boundaries- nurses must not overstep their duties by becoming intimate with patients. Nurses must also maintain professional relationships with their colleagues

The third provision: A nurse should assist and work for the well-being of the patient. This provision has six subdivisions:

1) Privacy
   - Nurses work to be sure patients have physical privacy by not allowing unwanted or unnecessary people into their room.
   - Nurses work to be sure patients have auditory privacy by not allowing confidential discussions to be overheard by others.

2) Confidentiality
   - Nurses work to maintain the patient's anonymity during consultations.
   - Nurses do not give information about patients to third parties except under strict protocols.
   - Nurses work to protect the patient's personal information.

3) Protection of participants in research
   - Patients have a choice when deciding about taking part in research.
   - Nurses make sure research subjects understand all information about the research.
   - Nurses make sure that research is conducted properly.
   - Nurses work to further the nursing profession through research.
   - Nurses work to implement research findings into practice.

4) Standards and review mechanisms
   - Nurses make sure that colleagues maintain professional work.
   - Nurses work to create new and improved policies in evaluation.
   - Nurses work to create better models for health care.

5) Acting on questionable practice
   - Nurses first question the individual who they believe may be acting improperly.
   - Nurses report any risk to patients to the proper authorities.
   - Nurses make sure that others follow the Code of Ethics.
   - Nurses should be protected from retribution when making reports of questionable practice.
6) Addressing impaired practice
   - Nurses should confront colleagues that are acting in ways that are not up to full standards
   - Nurses should be advocates for colleagues

The final three provisions of the Code of Ethics for Nurses with Interpretive Statements are:

- Provision Four: It is up to the individual nurse to be sure they are doing the best work possible.
- Provision Five: A nurse must be true to themselves and ethical in all actions.
- Provision Six: A nurse should make sure that the health care environment is as good as possible.
- Provision Seven: It is important to participate in continuing education.
- Provision Eight: A nurse works to advocate for their community.
- Provision Nine: It is the duty of nurses to maintain the professional standards of nursing practice.

Organ donation

The ethics of **organ donation** and transplants are decided upon by the Council on Ethical and Judicial Affairs (CEJA), which is part of the American Medical Association (AMA). These rules and regulations are constantly being revised and updated but one factor that is absolute is that all organs must be taken only on the consent of the donor or the person acting as the donor's legal advocate. The patient may state in a written document particular people or centers who should receive specific organs. If donation upon death is given without such stipulations then the United Network for Organ Sharing (UNOS) decides were the organs go based on the need of the patient and the time they were entered into the system. Organs that are donated by living donors are not regulated by a national system but by each individual transplant center. Usually living donors are relatives of the person they are donating too. However, the number of non-relative donations has increased dramatically in recent years due to news coverage and patient solicitation.

Pain relief and drug management

Relief from **pain** and the **management** of drugs used for pain is an ongoing ethical discussion within the medical field. Unfortunately, most patients do not receive appropriate relief from pain. It is the duty of the nurse to work with and on the behalf of patients and their pain management. The following are ideas for improving pain management.

- realize that medical care does not give patients the relief from pain that they need and merit
- assess the role of nursing in pain management
- be an advocate for patients who cannot stand up for their own rights
- explain to patients what forms of pain relief are available
- remember to see the patient as a whole not just as an illness
- stay abreast of the latest pain management techniques
- voice the problem of pain management to those around you including other health professionals, the public, etc
- work to change the systems and laws which make the management of pain relief so difficult

Managed care organizations and bioethics

There are several ethical conflicts between the use of managed care organizations (MCOs) and the principles of bioethics. The four principles of bioethics are:

autonomy, self-determination; beneficence, doing what is best for the patient; justice, all people receive the same level of care; social good, health care should be used for the common good. In order to gain the benefits of belonging to an MCO, patients and doctors have to give up some autonomy, as they no longer have complete freedom of choice. However, what are more troubling are the marketing practices, rules placed on doctors' freedom of speech, and management protocols used by MCOs. MCOs put making money above making people healthy. The MCO doctor gets a portion of profits, which can lead to them being less aggressive in their care of patients. By excluding individuals of a certain age or level of health from group plans MCOs violate the ethical principles of justice. Medicine as a social good has taken a huge hit with the creation of managed care. Many non-profit hospitals, teaching hospitals and programs, and research foundations have been purchased by MCOs who put profit above all else.

Ethical decision-making

A nurse has several resources to turn to when making ethical decisions. The American Nurses Association Code for Nurses and the American Hospital Association Bill of Rights are the documents that all nurses should know very well. The following methods will also guide nurses in their search for ethical solutions to difficult problems: a committee established to review co-worker decisions, the organization's rules on the use of technology, organization ethics committee that decides on the impact of new technology, and federal controls over limited resources. When a nurse is in doubt, asking the following questions may help him come to the appropriate answer: What historical knowledge can be applied to the presenting problem? What would be a solution everyone would be satisfied with? What may happen in the future is the solution is implemented?

Four Conservation Principles

Myra Levine developed Four Conservation Principles that are completely focused on the patient's welfare. In this model, the nurse has the ethical responsibility to treat each patient in a holistic manner that recognizes their individuality. With the information gained upon the patient's entry into the health care facility the nurse must create a plan of care that conserves the patient's energy, structural integrity, personal integrity and social integrity. **Conservation of energy** refers to keeping the patient at rest (heart rate low, blood pressure normal, temperature normal) in order to preserve the patient's resources for fighting the illness that brought them to seek care. These functions can be measured and recorded so that the patient's progress can be monitored consistently with the nurse making any necessary adjustments in care.

Principle two is termed the "**conservation of structural integrity** of the individual." Structural integrity refers to the body's natural state of health and well-being. Ethically a nurse should help a patient to return to normal using the best methods for that individual. A nurse must treat the entire person not only the illness, as when a person seeks health care it is not only the recuperation from illness that will return the person to their normal state. A nurse must be knowledgeable in Maslow's Hierarchy of Needs in order to help the individual regain self-esteem and self-confidence along with bodily health. Helping the patient to form goals and maintain health is very important to overall well-being.

Principle three is termed the "**conservation of personal integrity** of the individual." Personal integrity refers to a person's right to privacy. Maintaining an individual's privacy is a difficult problem in health care as the nurse must conduct physical assessments and ask the patient personal questions. However, a nurse can do these things in a manner that is respectful and sensitive to the patient's right to privacy. Principle four, the "**conservation of social** integrity of the individual", refers to a person's cultural interpretation of illness and coping methods. The nurse must understand that each patient comes from a unique background, which effects their social interactions. The nurse must respect these cultural differences and promote the patient's ties to their community.

Patient's Bill of Rights

There are eight categories described in the Patient's Bill of Rights developed by the President's Advisory Commission on Consumer Protection and Quality in the Health Care Industry. They are:

1) Information Disclosure: patients must be given information regarding all aspects of their health care in a way that is easy for them to understand.

2) Choice of Providers and Plans: patients must be allowed to choose between healthcare plans that are of high-quality.

3) Access to Emergency Services: patients must be allowed to go to an emergency room and have the bill paid for by their health care plan if they are in a severe situation and believe that if they don't get health care quickly they will be in serious jeopardy.

4) Participation in Treatment Decisions: patients or their guardians must be allowed to help make decisions about their treatment.

5) Respect and Nondiscrimination: patients must be treated with courtesy and consideration regardless of who they are, what they believe, etc.

6) Confidentiality of Health Information: patients must be able to speak to health care providers in private without fear that the information will be seen by non-essential parties. Patients must also be able to look at and photocopy their medical records upon request.

7) Complaints and Appeals: patients must be able to file complaints and have those complaints resolved in a fair and transparent manner. There must be both internal and external review systems of health care organizations.

8) Patient Responsibilities: patients must stand up for themselves and make an effort to be involved in their own health care.

Integrity

Integrity is defined by the American Heritage Dictionary as the "steadfast adherence to a strict moral or ethical code." Integrity is very important to nursing as without it there can be no bond of trust between nurse and patient. If it happens that a nurse is requested to perform a treatment or duty that is morally unacceptable to him then he may refuse the assignment on moral grounds. This refusal should if possible be given to management in written form well before the actual event occurs. However, if the event occurs with only the nurse present he must act in order to assure the patient's well-being.

The following situations may require the nurse to decide whether the action is ethical:

- Being asked to lie to a patient, change written data or withhold pertinent information

- Receiving verbal abuse from patients or colleagues

- Being told to act in a way that is different from the Code of Ethics for Nurses with Interpretive Statements

Healthcare Economics

Operating cycle

A health care organization that wants to survive in today's competitive market must act as a "going concern" developing and continuing an operating cycle. There are four stages in the operating cycle. First, the organization must define their mission statement according to the things they wish to achieve and the outside environment. Second, the organization must research whether or not its mission statement fits the needs and resources of the community. Third, resources must be packaged, priced, and offered to the community. Finally, the organization must be sure that enough money is made to balance out any money spent. Even if the first three steps are a success, an organization cannot run on a negative balance for very long. It may help to reassess charges for services or cut back on services that are very expensive to offer if the organization is not making a profit.

Income statements

There are two types of income statements used by managers to view profit and expense figures: external and management. External income statements are created to give a general overview of the company's finances or for people outside of the company to view. For health care organizations, external income statements generally include sales revenue; sale, administrative and general expenses; interest expense; income tax expense. Management income statements are created for nurse executives to get a broader picture of the company's finances. While the bottom line of both income statements is the same, the management income statement provides further details. This statement shows revenue by unit of sale, or in the case of health care, number of service hours or patients cared for. Another difference is that the management income statement divides expenses into two separate categories: variable and fixed.

There are many different accounting categories that can be found on an income statement. Sales revenue is the total amount of money made before any negating factors are taken into consideration. Gross margin is the figure found when subtracting costs from sales revenue. Inventory write-downs are a measure of money lost due to theft, damage, or expiration. Bad debts expense, also known as "write offs", is the money owed the organization that it will be unable to get back. Asset impairment write-downs include machines that need to be replaced or no longer work at 100% of their capacity. Depreciation expense is the cost of fixed assets over time as viewed as a fixed allocation of funds each year or estimated funds based on the assets' lifespan. Other sales, administrative, and general expenses that must be declared but do not fit into a specific category. Earning before interest and tax is money made minus expenses. Interest expense is money paid on debts. Income tax expense is money paid to federal and state governments. Net income is equal to all revenue minus all expenses.

Calculating profit

There are two methods for calculating an organization's profits: contribution margin minus fixed expenses and excess over breakeven volume x contribution margin per unit. Using the first method, total contribution margin is equal to the contribution margin per unit multiplied by unit sales volume. Earnings before interest and tax (EBIT), also called the operating profit, are found by subtracting total fixed operating expenses from the total contribution margin. Using the second method the breakeven point of sales must first be calculated. Then the contribution margin per unit is multiplied by the number of units sold in excess of the breakeven point to arrive at EBIT. This method subtracts fixed expenses, including interest, when calculating the breakeven point. It also calculates the organization's margin of safety, which is how much more was sold above the breakeven point.

Economies of scale

"Economies of scale" refers to the amount of output an organization can create based on its size. There are three categories of scale that an organization may experience as it grows. First, constant economies of scale are defined as an increase in scale percentage equal to the same increased percentage in output. For example, if a hospital increases the number of beds and personnel by fifty percent then it can service fifty percent more patients. Next, decreasing economies of scale are defined as an increase in size does not equal the same increase in output. This occurs when an organization becomes inefficient due to its large size. Finally, increasing returns to scale are defined as an increase in scale percentage realizes a larger increased percentage in output.

There are a number of reasons that very large companies enjoy enormous return to scale, also known as increasing economy of scale. First, capital intensiveness relates to the amount of money needed for success. In some businesses, oil and gas for example, start up costs are huge no matter if the company is large or small, but the high yield of a large company drives down the average fixed costs. Second, volume buying drives down the average variable costs. Next, administrative effectiveness includes both fixed and variable costs. For example, every organization, large or small, needs just one computer systems administrator, which is a fixed cost. As an organization grows it will need more computers, which is a variable cost, but this cost does not increase as quickly as output. Then, distribution includes both fixed and variable costs as well. Home health care workers receive an hourly salary (fixed cost) plus money for gas (variable). If they are able to see two patients who live in the same neighborhood this drives variable costs down. Finally, marketing power allows large companies to get their message across more easily and establish brand recognition further increasing their size.

Budgets

A budget is a plan on how to spend money on the various needs of an organization. Nurse administrators must make budgets in order to manage the financial resources of their organization. Managerial accounting shows how money is being used at the unit level. Financial accounting records how money is being made and spent. Assets are things of value such as cash, facilities and equipment. Liabilities are money owed by the organization. Revenue to money earned for services rendered. Generally, there are two types of centers in health organizations. Revenue centers charge the patient for their services. Types of revenue center include the pharmacy, operating room and lab. Cost centers do not charge the patient directly for their services but instead are paid for out of general hospital funds. Cost centers include housekeeping and maintenance.

There are three main types of budgets.
- Capital budgets take in account things that will need replacing or refurbishing such as buildings and are based on a three to five year plan.
- Cash budgets plan for the borrowing and investment of money depending on how much actual cash the organization believes it will need on hand.
- Operating budgets are based on a one to three year estimate, usually performed with the aid of a computer program that takes into consideration demand, operating costs and prices.

A more specific type of budget is known as the program/product line budget. These budgets look only at the unit level when deciding to highlight certain parts of the health organization.

Budgets are developed by looking at how much more or less should be spent in the coming year. It is necessary to try and determine areas that will need large upgrades in the near future so that the organization is not caught by surprise. Budgets also allow the monitor of how money is spent in relation to the effect is has on creating income. Budgets can also be used to motivate managers to handle their unit's money more carefully. When planning a budget it is important to communicate with other administrators in order to place the budget in the context of the larger organizational process. At times it may be necessary to justify an increase in the nursing budget by presenting research information or reports as to how the money will be effectively spent. Variance analysis can be helpful tool in finding problems in standards and performance.

Resource management

Resource management seeks to strike a balance between cost of care and quality of care. The development of a resource management system is done in three separate steps. First, as assessment is made. Depending on which resources are to be the emphasis of the developing plan an individual may look at past patient records including average level of illness, days in hospital and number of nursing hours utilized; the education and experience level of the health care providers; and what could happen if programs were changed. Next, a plan is developed. To develop a strong plan the ideas of staff and management should be solicited. Systems used by other health care organizations should also be reviewed. Finally, the plan is implemented. At this step a new budget must be created to match the plan. Implementation also includes keeping track of how the plan is going by receiving feedback from staff, patients and budget analysis.

Each resource management plan is created precisely for the environment into which it will be implemented but they all share the following basic principles.

- The first priority is always the patient.

- Quality workers must be on hand at all times.
- Teamwork is vital.
- Workers are appreciated.
- Nurses enjoy working in the same area for extended periods.
- Costs stay the same or go lower.
- Information is always being analyzed to make sure the plan is working well.
- The types of decisions an individual may make are obvious.
- Flexibility is key.

There are also several benefits that occur when resource management is successfully implemented. First, budgets are more balanced. Second, productivity gets better. Third, ideas to bring on new staff members are formed. Next, ideas for changing the way people work are formed. Finally, a set type of work evaluation is formed.

Staff management systems

GRASP, the Grace-Reynolds Application Study of PETO (Poland, English, Thornton, and Owens), is a system that assigns patients to units based on a mathematical formula that classifies the patients as they are admitted to the hospital. Another formula that works to balance number of patients by the number of nurses is the system developed by Chagnon, Audette, Lebrun, and Tilquin. Their formula states $P = (S + TUP)/360$ were "P" is the number of nurses, "S" is the time spent with patients, "TUP" are those things that nurses do on the job which are not classified under "S" and 360 is the time an individual nurse has to devote to "S" and "TUP". While both of these staff management systems deal with the raw number of nurses needed per patient they do not factor in the fact that some cases are more complex than others and therefore need a different mix of nurses.

Medicus Patient Classification System

One way to manage cost of care is to find the best ratio of nurses to patients. The Medicus Patient Classification System works by measuring how ill a patient is and therefore the number of hours of nursing care needed for him. Medicus is updated once every 24 hours to give the most accurate estimate possible. The nurse looks at such factors as level of consciousness, ability to care for self and pain level. The factors are scored and all points are added to determine the patient's illness level. A level I patient scores between 0 and 24 while a level VI, the most sick, may score up to 181 points. Medicus scores can be averaged for the entire unit in order to assign the appropriate number of nurses to each unit. Some health care organizations use the Medicus generated information to create budgets and plan future unit needs rather than making day to day changes in staff work.

Staff mix

Staff mix is the term used to describe the number of nurses holding certain degrees that work together. Because nurses who hold higher degrees are paid more than others, hospitals are trying to find an ideal balance between patient safety and care and costs. The nurses on a unit have a significant influence on how long patients stay in the hospital, the number of medical errors, how quickly nurses quit the service, and the rate of patient deaths. Often times health care organizations make decisions on staff mix based on patient classification systems (PCS). One main problem with using PCS is that inputting information into them takes away from the amount of time nurses have to actually care for patients and are not useful for short-term management. Other things that should be thought about when determining staff mix are how good the nurses are at their job, how difficult the work is, how the ward is organized, and what other staff members are on hand to help.

Productivity

Productivity is defined by the American Heritage Dictionary as "the rate at which goods or services are produced especially output per unit of labor." Productivity is represented by the mathematical formula $P=I/O$ where "P" is productivity, "I" is inputs and "O" is outputs. Inputs are any resources put into the system, money for example, while outputs are the amount of work provided by the system. Computer programs are sometimes used to find the best way to increase productivity. Some things that have been found to increase health care service productivity are: reducing the time a patient must wait to be seen by using a computerized scheduling system, restricting nurses to the areas they are most competent in, creating teams of health care workers from different specialties who work together to increase quality of patient care, and the study of ergonomics.

Healthcare Environment

Health care industry

As a whole, the health care establishment was the largest employer in the United States in 2004. There are nine categories in the health care establishment as defined by the U.S. Department of Labor. First, hospitals make up 1.9% of health care organizations, employee 41.3% of health care workers and provide diagnostic, inpatient, outpatient, emergency and long-term care. Second, nursing and residential care facilities make up 11.6% of health care organizations, employee 21.3% of health care workers and provide long-term inpatient care on a wide variety of levels. Next, physician's offices make up 37% of health care organizations, employee 15.5% of health care workers, provide diagnostic and preventative care and may work singly or in groups. Finally, dentist's offices make up 21% of health care organizations, employee 5.7% of health care workers and provide care for teeth.

Home health care services make up 3.0% of health care organizations, employee 5.8% of health care workers and provide diagnostic and preventative care in the patient's home. Second, outpatient care centers make up 3.2% of health care organizations, employee 3.4% of health care workers and provide wide variety of medical services such as "after hours" priority centers and kidney dialysis centers. Third, medical and diagnostic laboratories make up 2.1% of health care organizations, employee 1.4% of health care workers and provide blood analysis, x-rays and ultrasound exams. Next, other health practitioner's offices make up 18.7% of health care organizations, employee 4.0% of health care workers and include psychologists, dieticians and optometrists. Finally, other ambulatory health care services make up 1.5% of health care organizations, employee 1.5% of health care workers, provide transport services to hospitals and also include blood banks and organ donation establishments.

Consultations

The medical community is a good field to work in because no one really works alone but instead may call on a number of other professionals for advice and support. Consultation between nurses or with other health professionals should be encouraged. Nurses may wish to consult specialists during the formation of care plans in order to maximize the patient's treatment options while minimizing risk and cost. Nurses may be asked to consult because of specific skills they have or to educate patients on various tasks. There are six steps in the consultation process.

1) Decide what the problem is that needs to be addressed.
2) Find the right person for the particular problem.
3) Give the consultant any relevant information.
4) Do not give the consultant your opinion of the problem unless asked.
5) Be ready to listen to the consultants viewpoints.
6) Implement the advice given by the consultant.

Collaborative practice

There are six primary reasons why collaborative practice is more important in today's health service climate than ever before.

- There are more specialties that nurses can enter.
- The planning process often focuses on patient centered care.
- Nursing education does not always depict the reality of working as a nurse.
- Medical staff and management do not communicate enough.
- Increased focus on packaged health care services.
- Patients must be cared for over a broader spectrum of services.

When collaboration in a health organization works at high level there are many benefits to organization, patients and staff.

- more accurate diagnoses and fewer complications
- lowered anxiety levels and better understanding for family members
- emphasis on patient care before, during and after the hospital stay leads to better care overall
- less risk to patients due to treatment errors
- less money spent on consultation from outside sources

Interpersonal and professional relationships

Interpersonal relationships are close associations between two people. There are four stages in the formation of interpersonal relationships: contact, involvement, intimacy, deterioration, repair and dissolution. Some examples are friendship, marriage and coworker. An important part of how a person makes and sustains relationships is based on culture. As a nurse administrator, it is important to keep relationships with employees on a professional level. Depending on the formalness of the organization's environment and culture, this may include addressing employees by their title and last name, not discussing personal matters, being friendly but not making close friendships and not attending employees' private functions.

Analyzing organizational cultures

Often managers seek to study and analyze an organization's culture in order to better understand the inter-group relationships and to ease the process of organizational change. However, the ethical implications of such studies are often completely overlooked. First, information resulting from analyzing an organization's culture may be wrong. Culture is complex and impossible to completely assess. The analyst may place their own cultural values onto the information, which would further skew results. Next, once the organizations culture has been defined, individuals may feel pressured to change their work methods to match the organizations even when a change will not be positive for either party. Finally, some ethicists question the morality of administrators changing what their employees view as important or how they act. Employees have the right to maintain their personal culture.

Organizational structure

There are two main types of organizational structure: centralized and decentralized. Organizations that are managed using the decentralized method place more emphasis on the individual making decisions for themselves. While there is usually a management structure it is typically loosely based or lead positions are rotated among the staff members. For successful decentralization, each individual must know exactly what types of decisions they are free to make for themselves and which situations require input from an administrator or someone else in the chain of command. In very large organizations, separate units may be created which oversee themselves and therefore avoid a centralized manager who may favor some groups over others.

Along with decentralized, centralized organizational structure is one of the two main ways of managing health care facilities. A centralized organizational structure places greater decision making power in upper-level management. The administrative structure is rigid and obvious in its dealings with staff members. There are a great many reasons why organizations may wish to use a centralized organizational structure including: decisions are extremely important, lower-level leadership is week, and the facility is undergoing a rapid amount of significant change. Unfortunately, this management method usually misses out on the creativity and innovation of staff members as well as the risk that come by placing a lot of power into the hands of a single person.

Matrix organization

Matrix organization is one of the most recent models of management. There are three levels of administration within the matrix model.

1) top leader
   - Has power over the technical and administrative branches
   - Delegates authority
   - Shares responsibility for choices
   - Must be a very strong leader

2) matrix manager
   - Conducts worker performance evaluations
   - Makes day to day decisions on schedules and assignments
   - Follows unit goals

3) two-boss manager
   - Overseen by both the top leader and matrix manager
   - Must balance workers' needs with boss' wants

Committee structure

In very large organizations, responsibility for important functions may be divided into committees in order to maximize problem solving potential. Committees are overseen by a chairperson who guides meetings by a written agenda. Committee members discuss topics at length and then vote to form a consensus opinion. Typically one committee member takes notes, minutes, and is designated the secretary. There are five basic types of committees.

1) Governance: has the power to make decisions for the entire organization
2) Coordination: administrators from each unit of the organization meet to distribute resources, coordinate care, and define operation boundaries
3) Research and Recommendations: look into changing how the organization works

4) Project management: oversees defined projects ongoing within the organization

5) Specific committees: set up to perform clearly defined tasks such as creating budgets, overseeing health and safety, or ethics inquests

Governance model

"Governance model" means that the organization is under the control of a group of a governing board. The governing board works to protect the owners of the company, or in the case of a non-profit organization, the community. One of the main problems though is that board members are also likely to be working within the organization and therefore have a difficult time divorcing themselves from the need to protect worker interests, however in the end the governing board as a whole must work together for the owners' interests. While the board makes all decisions and is therefore the only one to blame when things go wrong they usually cannot fulfill their own demands without outside help. The board must be careful to choose staff that is highly proficient in their jobs.

Corporate culture

Corporate culture is defined as being the things which an organization finds important enough to use during the decision making process. The factors of corporate culture may be explicit, in the case of a mission statement, or implicit. In order to avoid conflict and maintain order it is important for the nurse administrator to understand their organization's corporate culture and make sure that all individuals have the same concept of what the important factors are. Corporate climate is defined as how the organization affects its workers. Some factors that influence corporate climate are the ways in which good employees are recognized, the amount and type of training that workers are given, communications processes and leader characteristics.

Shared governance model

The shared governance model of nurse administration states that no one individual is all powerful over a group of people. Instead, the shared governance model emphasizes that the entire group makes joint decisions and each individual is responsible for their work. In order to effectively use this model it is necessary that the organization adhere to a strict framework of administration.

- Each nurse must have an equal say about how their unit is run.
- Each individual should have a means to express their views on the overall running of the organization.
- Decisions regarding service must be made at the individual level.
- Nurses should understand that participation in organizational decision making is mandatory.
- A clearly defined mission statement must link the decisions made at each level of the organization.

Group formation

A group is a number of people working together toward a common goal. Groups work well because different people share their insight and creativity. Sometimes groups do not work well because individuals allow personal conflicts to interfere with the group's work. There are four stages to group development.

1) Forming
   - beginning of a group
   - individuals are quiet and polite
2) Storming
   - problems arise
   - not enough communication occurring

- 64 -

3) Norming
  - factions come together
  - communication flows more easily
4) Performing
  - group beings to really work
  - communication completely open

Team building

Team building refers to the creation of a collaborative group within the unit. When hiring new staff it is important to look for individuals who have personality characteristics that will blend well with existing employees and whose skills will fill a need within the unit. Bring the team together to form common goals, establish an internal leadership structure and assign specific roles to individuals. Support the team by helping them to clearly define goals and roles and moderate disputes. Give the team training in effective communication, conflict management and goal accomplishment. Reward team effort rather than recognizing an individual when goals are met. Finally, keep in close contact with the team in order to make sure that it is using resources properly and functioning as well as possible.

Conflict

According to Baldridge, there are four things that tend to cause conflicts. First, is the "iceberg phenomenon." In this situation a small problem unearths a deeper, larger problem. Second, is the idea that large problems bring people together in an effort to create a solution. Third, problems can happen when people want more than what they have currently. Finally, individuals may use ethical or moral issues to create conflict.

There are two basic types of conflict: intrapersonal and interpersonal. Intrapersonal conflict occurs only within the mind of the individual. This may happen because what the individual wants to be and what the individual actually is are very different things. Interpersonal conflict occurs between two people or groups. Nurse administrators should be well educated in conflict management, as this task will fall to them quite often.

When one individual is more powerful than another conflict is created between the two of them. There are five areas that will create conflict between a nurse administrator and the people she works with:

1) Reward power
   - being in a position to give achievement recognition
   - arises from being the one to hire and promote
2) Coercive power
   - being in a position to punish
   - arises from being the one to evaluate and fire
3) Legitimate power
   - held only by permission
   - must be a strong leader
4) Referent power
   - arises from the imitation of others
   - based on personality
5) Expert power
   - arises from knowing more than someone else
   - professional nursing knowledge
   - administrative skills

There are many ways to deal with conflict. First, is avoidance. Avoidance tries to act by not letting a situation become problematic. Avoidance is only useful if a fast solution can be enacted or if the situation is not very important. Second, is diffusion.

Diffusion works by placing the situation on a level of lower importance that it normally would be. Diffusion allows people space and time to calm down. This can be a helpful short-term solution. Third is containment. Containment controls a problematic situation by clearly defining what parts of the conflict will be talked about and how the problem will be solved. Finally, is confrontation. Confrontation faces the conflict head on. There are three types of confrontation. In a lose-lose situation both parties must give way to middle ground. In a win-lose situation one party is forced to back down by the other party. In a win-win situation, a solution is found that meets the needs of both parties.

Ethical conflicts

Nurses may find themselves involved in ethical conflicts with coworkers or supplementary personnel. It has been shown that individuals differ in their moral reasoning based on their educational level. Nurse administrators must be aware of this and ready for any conflicts that may arise as a result. Nurse administrators may also find that ethical issues occur when delegating work responsibility to other nurses. Nurses may also have ethical conflicts when working with physicians. First, nurses are paid by the hour while physicians are paid for services rendered. Physicians may want to admit more patients than a single nursing unit can comfortably handle. If nurses are overworked, they are more likely to make mistakes so it may be unethical for the physicians to over admit. Second, as advocates for the patient, nurses may feel at odds with a physician's decisions.

Professional Practice

Personnel policies

While every organization will have its own personnel policies and procedures there are some things that they will generally all have in common. First, each employee should have a personnel file with the following content: job applications, contracts, performance evaluations and disciplinary actions. An employee's I-9 forms and medical records should not be kept in their personnel file. Second, each organization should create an employee handbook outlining policies that pertain to every employee. These policies may include benefits, conflicts of interest, harassment, and paid holidays. Next, every organization should have an explicit disciplinary policy including the ways which disciplinary action should be documented. Finally, organizations should have standard evaluation methods for each unit or job description.

Communication

There are many different methods of communication. One element of communication that is often overlooked is **introspection**. Two elements of self communication are anger and revitalization. Often, individuals become angry on the job and because they cannot express that emotion in that context, their anger moves inward and can cause burnout and depression. Actively working to vent anger appropriately by writing the feelings down or communicating with the self in other ways is very helpful. Sometimes it feels as if everything is going wrong and the individual places blame upon themselves. In these times it is helpful to analyze the events and feelings in an objective manner so that revitalization can take place.

One-to-one communication is defined as two individuals taking turns listening and speaking to one another. Good administrators remember that listening is usually more important than speaking. It is a good idea to make regular meetings with staff members to discuss ongoing programs, problems, new ideas in the nursing field, and acting as a mentor. The nurse administrator should make sure that staff knows he is always there to help them work on problems. Another part of the regular meeting should be spent discussing the staff member's strengths and weaknesses being sure to commend the former and show ways to improve the latter. Conducting an interview is another time when nurse administrators must use one-to-one communication skills. In this case, it is important to make the applicant comfortable and to leave them with a positive view of the organization. This is done by preparing in advance what you will say.

There are ways to communicate: **verbally and nonverbally**. Verbal communication is either spoken or written. This form of communication can be either direct or indirect. Direct communication is those things that a person hears straight from the speaker. All other verbal communication can be edited and is therefore indirect. Fielden outlined five writing styles that can be used for different situations: forceful, passive, personal, impersonal and colorful. Nonverbal communication is all observable behavior. Examples of nonverbal communication include voice intonation, clothing, hand movements, facial expressions and the way the body is held. Approximately 90% of communication is received nonverbally so it is important to pay attention to nonverbal cues.

Persuasion and negotiation

Persuasion is a way of using communication to try to get someone to change their mind or behavior. Persuasion can only be achieved if the communicator knows the topic completely and has evidence to back up their claim. Negotiation is the strongest form of persuasion. The purpose of negotiation is to make all parties involved feel like they have won. The following are necessary if negotiation is to succeed: having a clear proposal, choosing the right day and time, using both written handouts and pictures to support the proposal, being aware of all verbal and nonverbal communication, and making the case known to the other party before negotiations begin. When getting ready to enter into negotiations there are three steps to complete in preparation. First, decide what you want and what you will settle for. Second, make yourself aware of how the other party feels. Finally, analyze external factors involved.

Interviewing

One of the jobs of the nurse administrator is to hire new staff. The following are examples of questions that can be used for the interviewing process. What process do you use to solve problems on the job? What makes you a good nurse? When feeling burn out what do you do? Have you ever had any problems with certain types of supervisors? If the head nurse asked you to do something you do not like to do, how would you respond? How do you cope with stress on the job? How long do you plan to stay in nursing? Did you ever think about being a doctor? How did you decide to become a nurse? How are you considerate of other's beliefs? What would you do if you were not a nurse? What type of people do you have a difficult time working with? Has anything on the job ever made you angry? How did you deal with it? How do you make decisions?

Nursing research

Some organizations place an emphasis on conducting research. In order for research to be begun easily, the following factors should be in place. First, the nurse administrator must have knowledge and experience in conducting research. Second, there must be support from staff members. Finally, the organization must be fully committed to backing nursing research with appropriate support and funding. There are five different models for nursing research programs.

- University-based model: research started by professors at nursing school, typically takes place in a lab- reported in peer-reviewed journals
- Agency-based model: organization brings in research professionals to lead in-agency research- nurses play a large part in conducting the research Collaborative university:-agency based model, one person heads a team at a university and a at a separate health care facility- combines information from both areas.
- External consultant model: organization hires a professional researcher for one particular study- nurses provide researcher information.
- Nursing development unit model: educates unit nurses to conduct research within their area; allows nurses to be published in peer-reviewed journals

Nursing units and research

In order to advance nursing as a profession, it has become necessary for nurses to conduct research and put the findings from research into practice. There are several areas where research findings can be easily put into the service of a nursing unit or nurse administrator. The first is changing the number of nurses on duty and the number of hours they work in a shift. The second area that research findings can impact is how well the patients feel they are being treated. Finally, evaluation of care models can be affected by research data. One model of research that can be used by nursing units is participatory action research. Not only does this model lead to finding new ways to work but also strengthens those groups who participate in it. The research design should be simple enough that all unit nurses can take part in every stage with the results being self explanatory. If necessary, an outside professional researcher may be brought in to lead the team and teach the necessary research skills. Professionals in other areas such as computer technology or strategic planning may also be utilized.

Community epidemiology studies

Community epidemiology is the study of diseases and illnesses that occur in pre-defined locations. Community epidemiology is closely linked to public health advocacy as often researchers may find environmental links between the illness and community. There are three types of studies used to research community epidemiology. First, are case-series studies. Case-series studies give an in-depth report on one person but the information cannot be generalized to the entire community. Second, case control studies group people into two categories: those who have the disease and those who do not have the disease. Comparisons are made between the two groups based on what the subjects say happened. This type of study is subject to memory fallibility. Finally, prospective studies, also known as cohort studies, observe people who are healthy but have different habits that the researcher wishes to learn about. This type of study takes a long time and may cost a lot of money as the subjects are observed for many years.

Human subjects in clinical trials

All research that intends to use human subjects must be submitted to a review board before any actions can begin. The review board should also be available to hear subject complaints, review research in progress and investigate alleged subject abuse. The National Commission of the Protection of Human Subjects of Biomedical and Behavioral Research produced the first set of legislation regarding the use of human subjects in clinical research. The Belmont Report outlined three basic ethical principles.

1) Respect for individuals.
   - people must give informed consent
   - informed consent consists of understand information regarding the study
   - all subjects must be volunteers

2) Kindness to individuals.

- people should not be hurt physically or mentally
- maximize benefits- minimize risk

3) Fairness to all participants.

- random selection of subjects
- random grouping into categories

AHRQ

The United States Public Health Services Agency for Healthcare Research and Quality (AHRQ) supports evidence-based Practice Centers, which develop and publish their ideas for managing healthcare. The evidence-based Practice Centers (EPCs) are charged with the task of analyzing all applicable scientific findings in one or more of the following categories: clinical, behavioral, and organizing and finance. The reports generated are then used to guide policy decisions in healthcare administration. For example, a report on literacy rates may change the type of educational materials used with certain populations. The main goal of AHRQ and its EPC partners is to improve the caliber, capability and consistency of healthcare. The reports are extremely specific and exact about what methods were used, give explanations as to why the methods were chosen and ideas into why the methods work. A number of statistical methods including meta-analysis and cost analysis are used in interpret the data.

Retention and turnover considerations

Due to a critical shortage of nurses, recent emphasis has been place on retention and turnover problems. Recruiting uses an organization's valuable resources at a higher rate than retaining those nurses already employed. One of the biggest factors in turnover is how the organization's administration interacts with the employees. The following factors are also often stated as reason's why nurses quit: small number of nurses who are good leaders or part of the management, not being paid enough and slow promotion, poor public image, too much responsibility in comparison to admiration, problematic shift work, too much overtime work necessary, poor treatment by doctors, educational level higher than work being asked to do, inability to make decisions, being overworked, not being able to do a good job because too much work, being moved into areas of inexperience, no support from organization.

Recruitment

With today's shortage of nurses, health care organizations must find new ways to bring in top quality employees. Focusing on the organization's mission statement and marketing it is one way to attract nurses. Agreeing to take over student loan payments and offering sign-on bonuses and promotion focused positions can also be effective. Also, remember to ask current employees to refer their friends to the organization. Be sure that job descriptions identify the best things about being a nurse and include comments from current employees about what a fantastic place it is to work. Know what other health organizations are doing to recruit and retain staff then do more. Concentrate recruitment advertising in the areas that current employees recommend.

Ethical recruitment of international nurses

Due to the shortage of nurses that increased during the 1990's health care organizations began intensive recruitment of foreign nurses in the early part of the 21st century. The National Council of State Boards of Nursing has gone on record as supporting the need for legal immigrant nurses to work in the U.S. but has also stated a number of factors that must be dealt with. First, standards for international nurses practicing in the U.S. must not be lowered. Second, international nurses should have to pass an English language exam before receiving a license to practice. Third, criminal background checks should be run within the U.S. and internationally.

Next, international nurses need to have the same pass score on licensure tests as U.S. nurses. Finally, the shortage issue needs to be dealt with in more proactive ways than simply importing nurses.

The shortage of American nurses has led to the recruitment of nurses internationally. The National Council of State Boards of Nursing has issued statements regarding ethical practices in internal recruitment and standards. Not only must recruitment organizations abide by the normal ethical rules for hiring practices but should also include the following five practices.

1) Any work offer made to the international nurse should not contain hidden traps or false information.
2) International nurses must be given the chance to make an informed decision by having available information about living and working conditions, immigration laws, and work environment.
3) Recruiters must inform the prospective employee about licensure rules and regulations.
4) All recruiters must adopt high ethical standards.
5) Recruiters who do not act ethically should be punished in some way.

Job satisfaction theories

Job satisfaction is defined by how happy an individual is on the job. Affect theory was developed by Edwin A. Locke and satisfaction is stated as the difference between what an individual wants on the job and what they actually have on the job. Those things about the job that are most important to the individual will have the most influence on their level of satisfaction. Dispositional theory states that it is the individual's internal amount of satisfaction that has the largest effect as to whether they are happy on the job. The Core Self-Evaluations theory outlines four personality characteristics that influence a person's job satisfaction. These characteristics are self-esteem, self-efficacy, locus of control, and neuroticism.

Finally, Motivator Hygiene theory, states that motivators are things that make a person want to work and hygiene are those things that make a person unhappy on the job.

Labor laws

There are two types of general labor laws: collective and individual. Collective labor laws are those statutes that govern the dealings between employer, employee and union. Trade (labor) unions are formed to protect the employees' rights under these laws. Unions have several methods by which they can force a company to negotiate with them or bend to their viewpoint. First, union employees may strike. In a strike, employees refuse to come to work. Second, when unions are not allowed to strike legally they may perform a "sickout" which occurs when a large percentage of employees call in sick, often stating they have "the flu". Finally, striking employees may form picket lines in an attempt to keep other workers from entering the place of employment.

Individual labor law deals with a person's rights on the job and their personal contract with the employer. With the increasing education level of American workers and the tightening of collective labor laws less responsibility is being placed on unions and is instead being transferred to the individual worker. Individual labor laws include equal opportunity, minimum wage, amount of break time, sexual harassment, and unfair dismissal. Equal opportunity is those laws that prohibit employers from denying work to an individual due to sex, religion, race, etc. Minimum wage is the lowest amount an employer can pay a worker. Typically an employer must provide a morning and afternoon break plus a period for lunch during the workday. Sexual harassment refers to pressuring an individual with sexual advances. All employees have the right to dispute their actions before being fired.

Fair Labor Standards Act

The Fair Labor Standards Act of 1938 (FLSA) has been amended several times to set standards for minimum wage, child labor and other employment guidelines. The current federal minimum wage is $7.25 per hour with a minimum of "time and a half" for work done over 40 hours a week. Individual states may have higher minimum wages than the federal set limit. The minimum working age is 16 but may be lowered with exceptions. The FLSA also forbids discrimination in employment and pay on the basis of sex, age, religious beliefs, disability and sexual orientation. The FLSA is overseen by the United States Department of Labor and more specifically the Wage and Hour Division, which may bring lawsuits against employers on behalf of the employees.

National Labor Relations Act

The original National Labor Relations Act was signed into law as the Wagner Act in 1935. This act made it illegal for employers to treat employees unfairly and created the National Labor Relations Board, which looks into charges of unfair treatment and holds elections for non-union employees on the issue of becoming unionized. In 1947, the Act was amended by the Taft-Hartley Act, which placed restrictions on unions. In particular, the Taft-Hartley Act made it illegal for union workers to strike in the following situations: work assignment issues or as part of a secondary boycott. It also became illegal for unions to require companies to hire only union workers and gave power to individual states regarding some union policy.

Equal Employment Opportunity Commission

The Equal Employment Opportunity Commission enforces laws that prohibit job discrimination. Title VII of the Civil Rights Act of 1964 "prohibits employment discrimination based on race, color, religion, sex or national origin." The Equal Pay

Act of 1963 requires employers to pay men and women the same amount of money for jobs which are the same or highly similar. People who are older than 40 are protected against discrimination in the workplace by the Age Discrimination in Employment Act of 1967. Title I and Title V of the Americans with Disabilities Act of 1990 prevents employers in both the private sector and state and local governments from discriminating in the hiring of people with disabilities. The federal government is also not allowed to discriminate against people with disabilities according to Sections 501 and 505 of the Rehabilitation Act of 1973. Finally, the Civil Rights Act of 1991 allows individuals to receive money if they are discriminated against.

Affirmative action

Affirmative action is the idea that because some groups of people have been discriminated against in regards to hiring and pay these groups should be given preferences in hiring today. These groups include, women, African Americans and people with disabilities. In some cases, the preferences may come in the form of quotas, meaning that a certain percentage of employees must come from minority groups. Another form of preference gives points to prospective employees based on their membership in certain minorities. Recently there has been a backlash against affirmative action claiming that it is merely another form of discrimination. Some states have considered repealing affirmative action laws but until otherwise informed an administrator should continue to follow all affirmative action regulations.

Contract negotiations

Once a labor union and a company have formed a contract, it is up to the company's managers to make decisions on daily operating procedure and discipline. There are many issues in contract administration that can lead to problems for managers. These include:

- Discipline: how bad behavior is dealt with
- Incentives: the way bonuses are awarded
- Work Assignments: job definitions and role clarification
- Individual Personnel Assignments: how employees are promoted, given shift work, etc.
- Hours of Work: standard schedules and over-time pay
- Supervisors Doing Production Work: job security
- Production Standards: amount of work an individual is given
- Working Conditions: concerns over health, safety, and comfort
- Subcontracting: brining in non-union workers
- Past Practice: continuing historical precedents
- Rules: creation of new policies not in contract

All legally binding contracts have the following eight features.

1) Terms: defines what the parties are agreeing to do
2) Mutual Agreement: proof that all parties have agreed to the terms
3) Consideration: one party must gain something while the other party looses something
4) Competent, Adult Parties: individuals who enter into contracts must have the mental capacity to understand the terms of the contract
5) Proper Subject Matter: contracts can only be made for things that are legal
6) Mutual Right to Remedy: if a violation of contract is made by one party then the other party can attempt to fix the problem through legal means
7) Mutual Obligation to Perform: all parties must keep their promises
8) Intention to Create Legal Relationship: similar to "good faith" agreements, both parties must enter the contract with lawful intentions

Generally there are three main ideas used to create contracts. One idea is offer and acceptance. An offer is a statement that a party wishes to enter into a contract with another party. An offer may be stated orally, implied or written as in a letter, newspaper, or email. A "unilateral contract" occurs when the party expected to accept the contract completes the expected action without formal acceptance. An "invitation to treat" is not the same as an offer but is instead a sign that an individual would like to make a bargain. The individual who makes an offer may revoke it at any time before it is accepted as long as the other party is informed.

Acceptance occurs when both parties agree to the terms of a contract. There are six generally accepted rules that relate to the announcement of acceptance.

1) agreement to the contract must be announced in some form otherwise the offering party has the right to withdrawal the offer

2) a contract can only be agreed to by the individual to whom the offer was made

3) if an individual agrees to a contract for someone else without their consent then the person is not legally bound to the contract

4) the wording of a contract may include the insinuation that the individual has announced agreement to the contract

5) if the way in which the offer should be accepted is stated in the contract the individual who is accepting must use that method or its equivalent

6) a failure to reply is not the same as agreement

One idea used in the creation of contracts is known as consideration and **estoppel**. Common law and civil law treat the concept of consideration differently. Common law states that each party must give something to make the contract legally binding. Civil law states that one party may give something to another party without receiving something in return. Estoppel is the idea that if a person makes a promise to someone else they cannot later change their mind if the person they promised to was relying on that promise.

Another idea used in the formation of contracts is the intention to be **legally bound**. This refers to both parties entering into a contract with the notion that the terms are mandatory.

Collective bargaining

Collective bargaining is a method used by unions and managers to come to an agreement on problems. Interest disputes that occur when a union and a company's managers cannot agree on basic employment issues are often settled with collective bargaining. There are two sub-types of collective bargaining. First, pattern bargaining occurs when a large union tries to carry over an agreed plan from one company to another. For example, a union representing nurses in the state of California might try to get Hospital B to accept the contract specifics of Hospital A. Centralized bargaining is used when either the union or employer wishes to combine appropriate bargaining units to facilitate the bargaining process. Centralized bargaining is further split into two types. Single employer-multiplant bargaining is often used when a company has several manufacturing facilities which are interdependent. Multiemployer bargaining is often used when there are many different companies that have the same type of employee such as professional basketball teams.

There are two dimensions in the ethics of collective bargaining. The first dimension, moral or ideal behavior, can be hard to quantify. There are some things that are absolutely wrong such as using bribes, stealing proprietary information, and attempting to listen in on meetings using electronic surveillance equipment. The second dimension, conforming to professional standards can be broken down into three generally agreed on standards that the representative should possess. 1) Getting what their group needs for the agreement. 2) Showing their coworkers and group members that they have good negotiating skills. 3) Communicating with the other group in a way that makes the process easier and leaves the door open for future settlements. Some issues that have an ethical imperative are also back up with laws. One such issue is "good faith bargaining" which states that offers are made that if agreed upon will be enacted.

Grievances

Employees or union representatives may file a grievance when they feel that the employer has done something contrary to the company's policies or labor agreement. There are four general reasons why grievances may be filed. First, a grievance may be filed to protest a contractual violation. This may happen when a circumstance occurs that is not explicitly spelled out in the labor agreement and management exercises its right to form a decision. Second, a grievance may be filed to draw attention to a problem in the work environment. This may happen when an individual is concerned about a safety issue or the union wants to highlight a problem they wish to include in future negotiation proceedings. Third, a grievance may be filed to make the employee and/or union feel important. This may happen when an employee feels that a manager is being too pushy or authoritarian or when union elections are approaching. Finally, a grievance may be filed to get something for nothing. This may happen when an employee sees a situation that he can exploit to his advantage.

The majority of labor unions have a three step procedure for dealing with employee grievance claims, however some may include a fourth step as well. The first step is broken down into two parts. First, the employee talks to their manager about the problem. If the employee and manager cannot reach a conclusion then the employee files a written statement. The supervisor responds also in writing. Once a conclusion is made, it is unnecessary to continue the grievance process. In step two, low level union representatives enter the process. In step three, higher level union officials become involved. In step four, the problem is given over to an arbitrator or mediator.

EAP

An employee assistance program (EAP) is a source of help for employees or certain family members in specific situations. Providing employee counseling through an EAP is an excellent way of retaining staff. Also, better adjusted staff make fewer on the job errors and have fewer absences form work. Although EAP counseling is generally held on site, patient-client confidentiality is still maintained. Individual EAP counseling may include mental, family, marriage, stress, finances or addiction counseling. EAP counselor may also give "brown-bag" seminars that employees are encouraged to attend on their lunch hour covering topics on both professional and home life situations.

Orientation

Orientation is an essential part of keeping employees happy and informed from the start. Orientation can be made up of relaxed times when new nurses are allowed to meet one another under little pressure and formal training times. The following are ideas to keep in mind during orientation. Present the organizational mission statement, history and goals. Allow employees to complete tax information and other paperwork. Explain the employee benefits. Give parking permits or other necessary permits. Discuss infection control measures. Hold a fire drill. Introduce the computer system. Demonstrate proper wound care. Present the dress code. Discuss and practice safe and appropriate use of restraints. Give a complete tour of the facilities. Discuss guidelines for working around blood. Outline promotion tracks. Examine risk management. Practice using equipment. Introduce management personnel.

Continuing education and training

The health care system in which nurses work is constantly changing due to the rapid advances in medicine and technology. Continuing education must be a part of every nurse's professional life as what she learned in school a few years ago may be completely out of date now. Also, depending on which state the nurse practices in, continuing education may be required by law. Continuing education usually takes place over the course of a weekend seminar but may also consist of semester long classes at a local educational institution. In-service training takes place within the health care organization and is usually done during normal working hours. This training typically focuses on changes that will be taking place with the organization, issues of health and safety or policy clarification.

Re-educating staff nurses

Since the inception of nursing as a career it has been based in hospital organizations and treating the patients there. Now due to the rise in health care costs as well as new treatments, such as outpatient surgery, which require far shorter hospital stays, the field of nursing is turning to other venues for delivery of care. Even within the hospital environment, nursing duties have been scaled back or changed so dramatically that it is often difficult for nurses who have been working in the field more than twenty years to adapt. It is extremely important that nurse education systems be overwhelmed at every level. The nurse administrator must take on the job of re-educating staff nurses in order to ensure high quality care for patients, high retention rates of qualified nurses and lower costs.

Employee recognition

Employee recognition is an important part of a nurse administrator's job. Recognition makes people want to work harder, do better and stay on the job. In order for recognition to be successful, there are a number of things that should be done. First, no employee should be ineligible for recognition. Second, the process of recognition should be clearly outlined. Third, be sure to let employees know exactly why they are being recognized. Next, do not wait too long between the admirable work and the recognition. Also, allow the employees to have some input in who is recognized. Do not allow recognition to appear to be an entitlement. Try to make random days fun or interesting so that the entire staff feel recognized and appreciated.

Performance evaluation

<u>Rating scales</u>

A method of performance appraisal that seeks to look only at the work an employee is doing is called **Behaviorally Anchored Rating Scale** (BARS). BARS does not look at the employee's disposition or personal character. A BARS is typically created by management for a specific unit or job description. First, the job is analyzed and lists of specific necessary behaviors are drawn up. Next the behaviors are categorized. Finally, a scale is made up for each category. Each point along the scale, poor, good, excellent is defined specifically so that both employee and rater know exactly what is expected. BARS was created to be a better alternative to graphic ratings scales, but to date research has not shown BARS to be worth the extra effort involved in scale creation for use in most situations.

Graphic rating scales (GRS) are a very easy to create and use system of performance appraisal. In fact, an organization may be able to pick from a wide variety of pre-produced GRS to use rather than creating their own saving time and other resources. GRS are not particularly in depth but they are very reliable. The GRS list a number of work behaviors, for example, "Arrives at work on time." and usually some personal characteristics as well, "Greets patients in a friendly manner." for example. It is up to the rater to circle the answer which best describes the employee. The answer scale is usually, "outstanding, above average, average, poor, and unsatisfactory" or something similar. There are two main problems with GRS. First, each person may define "average" differently leading the rater and employee to a different assessment of the appraisal. Second, unless notes are added in explanation the employee may not understand why they were given a "poor" rating nor know how to improve.

Assessments

Peer review performance appraisal is used to set unit goals and create a co-operative atmosphere of reaching goals and working harder. This type of assessment should not be used as a basis of promotion, disciplinary action or pay. Generally, several workers form a team to assess their colleagues on a rotating schedule giving each employee a chance to be reviewed and to review. 360-degree feedback combines several different types of performance appraisals so that a wide picture of organizational function can be obtained. 360-degree feedback fosters the risk of personal bias and discrimination. Unfortunately, 360-degree feedback tends to focus on weaknesses and takes a lot of organizational resources to create.

Progressive discipline

Progressive discipline is a means to let employees know they are not working at an expected level. Discipline is not the same as punishment but instead a chance for the employee to improve. There are five basic steps to progressive discipline.

1) Talk to the employee about what is necessary to do a good job and how they can do better.
2) Give the employee a verbal admonition.
3) Place a reprimand in the employee's file and let them know you have done so.

4) Place the employee on suspension. Start with one day of suspension and if the employee does not improve increase the number days, one at a time, up to five.

5) Fire the employee if they cannot or will not get better.

Ladder of advancement

Nurses have many opportunities for advancing within their field. In the past nurses had to return to school in order to receive a higher educational level to then advance on the job. Now organizations often use career, sometimes referred to as clinical, ladders to define the exact process an individual must take to achieve promotion. This allows the nurse to benefit because she is able to work while advancing to more responsibility but perhaps has even more benefits for the health care organization as it allows them to promote "in-house" and increases their retention rates. There are several paths individuals can take within an organization including administration, research and education. One of the most important parts of presenting a career ladder to employees is that each factor of the promotion process be completely defined and transparent. Employees should be encouraged to use both self-review and peer-review for feedback in the ladder procedure.

Motivators

Motivators can be defined as those things that influence a person's desire to act. Herzberg outlined internal and external factors that can work as motivators. External factors include management style, pay, what happens away from work, whether or not the individual feels secure in their job, work environment, and organization policies. Internal factors include reaching goals, promotion, recognition, job satisfaction, personal growth, and amount of responsibility. David McClelland saw motivation in a slightly different way. McClelland outlined three things that work to motivate all people: the desire to reach goals or perform above average, the desire to influence other people's behavior, and the desire to have personal relationships on many levels.

Job enlargement and enrichment

Job enlargement can be defined as horizontal promotion as it gives an employee more duties without an increase in pay. Job enrichment increases the employee's happiness with their work by making it more interesting or rewarding. There are three stages involved in job enrichment.
1) Amount of effort should be visible in the quality of the performance.
   - make teamwork essential
   - let every individual know their place in the organization
   - give regular feedback
2) Give rewards based on performance.
   - Define quality performance
   - use explicitly defined reward
3) Let employees choose rewards by giving surveys or holding meetings on the subject.

Roles of nurses

Nurses serve many roles within the framework of caring for patients. The following seven examples give an overview of what nurses do in their profession.
1) Care Giver: provides medical treatment and works with the patient to set goals
2) Protector and Client Advocate: keep patient safe, works to prevent injuries and protects the patient's ethical rights
3) Manager: bring various health care workers together for treatment of the patient, looks after own career, uses time wisely

4) Rehabilitator: helps patients function as completely as possible

5) Comforter: listens to patients and helps them complete goals

6) Communicator: speaks clearly to patients, family members and other health care workers

7) Teacher: helps patients understand what is happening and helps family learn to care for the patient

Advanced nursing careers

Nurses have more opportunity for developing specialized careers than ever before. The nurse educator works primarily in schools of nursing teaching students to become nurses themselves. Nurse educators may also work in health care organizations teaching patients specifics about illness and how to care for themselves. Clinical nurse specialists hold a master's of nursing and have done fieldwork to specialize in a specific area of practice such as community health, geriatrics or cardiology. There have been large increases in the number of nurse practitioners in the past twenty years. Nurse practitioners may take the place of a primary care physician in treating patients in health clinics. The certified nurse-midwife (CNM) works with women during pregnancy, childbirth and the post-natal period. A CNM does not need to work with a medical physician. Finally, nurse anesthetists work with anesthesiologists during surgery.

Alternative-care settings

While the majority of nurses are employed by hospitals, there are several **community alternative-care settings** where they may choose to work as well. Community health clinics provide basic services such as birth control advice and well baby check-ups. Nurses are the main caregivers in such facilities and therefore have more freedom than nurses in hospitals. Schools hire nurses to teach health education classes, be on hand for non-emergency problems and to perform annual eye and hearing checks. Nurses working for private companies may give lectures on improving health and safety, keep on top of OSHA guidelines, provide first aid and provide emergency care while waiting for other health care professionals to arrive. The health care service set to see the largest growth in the near future is home health care agencies. Nurses may perform routine tasks such as dispensing medications, giving i.v. therapy and wound care or take on the role of educator to instruct family members.

Due to the rise in health care costs, several **alternative-care institutional settings** have arisen to manage health services. Extended care facilities become more numerous every year due to the ageing of the American population. There are two different types of extended care facilities: intermediate care and long-term care. Intermediate care facilities exist to help patients who no longer need the round the clock care of a hospital but are not well enough to go home either. Long-term care facilities are generally, for older adults who need help with daily life functioning more than medical services. There are also two main types of rehabilitation centers that help individuals in a residential setting. Physical rehabilitation centers work with people who have developed a problem in their ability to physically function. Drug rehabilitation centers work to get people off drugs and stay drug free.

Nursing qualifications

There are several levels of education nurses can obtain to work within the health care field. Certified nursing assistants (CNAs) work under the supervision of more senior nurses helping patients with eating, dressing, walking and other activities and provide basic medical services like giving medications and taking blood pressure readings. To achieve the title CNA, individuals must complete 75 hours of nursing education including 16 hours of on-the-job training. Licensed practical nurses (LPNs) must also work under the supervision of an upper level nurse. LPNs generally have a two-year degree and must pass the National Council Licensure

Examination (NCLEX) in order to receive work permission. LPNs may work in hospitals or private clinics. Registered nurses (RNs) oversee the work of CNAs and LPNs in addition to caring for patients. RNs may have a bachelor's degree and must pass the NCLEX-RN to practice.

Magnet Recognition Program®

The Magnet Recognition Program® was created to find and promote health care organizations that have a very good nursing staff. The program was created by the American Nurses Credentialing Center. Nursing staff are judged qualitatively and quantitatively according to the Scope and Standards for Nurse Administrators written by the American Nurse's Association. When choosing a health care facility, patients can look for the programs seal of approval and know they will be provided with the very best nursing care possible. Newly graduated nursing students may also wish to look for Magnet Recognition Program® recognized facilities so they can be sure to join a good job environment. The program places an emphasis on nurses in leadership positions and continuing education in the workplace.

Certification

The American Nurses Credentialing Center (ANCC) provides advance practice certification for nurse practitioners, clinical nurse specialists, nurse administrators, and diabetes dietician and pharmacy management. The ANCC also offers a wide variety of specialty certification. Certification is determined by a test and is good for five years. Renewal of certification can be accomplished by providing proof of 1,000 hours of practice or retest. Certification shows that the nurse has a thorough understanding of their specialty according to national standards.

There are many other certification boards that give nurses certification in various specialties. For example, the National Certification Corporation certifies nurses in obstetrics and gynecology positions.

National Council Licensure Examinations

The National Council of State Boards of Nursing create and administer the National Council Licensure Examination (NCLEX) for Registered Nurses (-RN) and for Practical Nurses (-PN). The NCLEX is a computerized adaptive test, which means that each individual will receive different levels and numbers of questions depending on how many correct answers they give. The NCLEX-RN test taker will have to answer at least 75 questions and a maximum of 265 while the NCLEX-PN test taker will have to answer at least 85 questions and a maximum of 205. A maximum of five hours is allowed for the exam. Both exams ask questions on the following content: safe effective care environment, health promotion and maintenance, psychosocial integrity and physiological well-being. The NCLEX must be passed before a nurse has the right to work in the profession.

Self-assessment

Self-assessment is a performance appraisal tool that can be used with other types of management appraisals or by itself to help an individual analyze their past performance and develop goals for future self-improvement. For successful self-assessment the following practices should be done. First, self-assessment should be performed regularly. Next, the job should be broken down into aspects of technical, administrative, and communication. The individual may then use a rating scale to rate their performance on a number of factors within these categories. Nurse administrators may rate themselves on their use of new budgeting software, making subordinate work schedules, and how well they are keeping upper management informed of the nurse retention problem. Finally, the results of each self-assessment should be written out and reviewed regularly in order to stay on track.

Nurse administrator role

Nurse administrators do not look after patients or give direct health care but instead manage the nursing department. It is the nurse administrator's job to act as a link between the nurses and the organizational management. They also create budgets, work to secure resources and create strategic plans. It is important for nurse administrators to follow the ethical guidelines set for them by the American Nursing Academy and to treat all staff with respect regardless of their background. They may work to hire and keep staff nurses, delegate tasks, resolve conflicts between nurses and between the nursing department and the organization. Nurse administrators may also supervise student interns; collaborate with colleagues to create a care environment that is high quality and low cost. They also perform research and apply research findings to current practice.

Contingency models of leadership

There are three contingency models of leadership. However, autocratic-democratic, which only defines two extremes, is not very good in the various situations in which a nurse administrator works. On the other hand, the Fiedler model is based on three dimensions. The leader-member relations dimension defines the relationship between the workers and the administrator. The task structure dimension defines what type of work the administrator gives to the employees. The position power dimension defines how much the leader is able to change factors of power. The main idea behind the Fiedler model is that the personality of the leader effects how the workers perform. In contrast, path-goal theory is based on the idea that the personalities of the workers effects how the leader performs. When using the path-goal theory of leadership it is very important to keep open the lines of communication between subordinates and managers and to allow the ideas of the subordinates to direct the way in which problems are solved.

Continuum-based leadership model

The continuum-based leadership model, also known as the model for the year 2000, is based on the idea that organizations work in ways that are similar to quantum functioning in that there is no top or bottom but only the whole with individuals moving fluidly in and out of leadership roles as the situation demands. This model calls for an end to the single all powerful nurse administrators replaced by a number of administrators taking up specific lines of administrative functioning. The administrators must then work on behalf of their subordinates in the appropriation of resources and must work together with their colleagues to ensure the fair and reasonable distribution of those resources. The continuum-based model also places emphasis on all "nurse executives" obtaining leadership skills as their job satisfaction with being overseen by a true leader.

Management styles

There are four basic styles of management: autocratic, democratic, consultative and laissez-faire. Democratic managers strive to empower their employees by giving them responsibility. Employees are crucial to decision making when democratic leadership is applied. Autocratic managers tell their employees exactly what they must do and how to do it. While autocratic management leads to the ability to make quick decisions it also tends to alienate employees. Consultative managers ask for employees' views and thoughts but make decisions by themselves. Laissez-faire, also known as permissive, managers allow employees to make nearly all decisions on their own. The primary task in laissez-faire management is to answer questions and serve as a guide to employees.

Classical management

The theory of classical management places all emphasis on the manager's ability to find solutions for their workers. In turn, workers perform well due to the desire for financial security. While there have been many people who explored classical management theory they all agree that there are three steps in the management process: planning, organizing, and controlling. Fredrick W. Taylor founded the science of management and believed that managers and their workers should cooperate and share responsibility. The Gnatt chart developed by Henry L. Gnatt compares work desired/work finished to time of completion. Frank and Lillian Glibreth studied people at work in order to find the best and most efficient way for work to be done. Similarly, Henri Fayol, working in France, developed ideas for creating efficient and capable managers.

Organizational development model

The organizational development model (OD) of change within an organization works by focusing on the culture of the organization. OD encourages management worker cooperation and communication and its primary goal is to make the workplace a good environment for everyone. There are several steps that must take place in order for OD to be beneficial. First, the dynamics of the organization are studied and accurately described. Next, a comprehensive plan for problem solving should be carried out. Finally, resources are bought and the plan is put into place. These three comprehensive steps can be further broken down into the following: initial diagnosis, data collection and confrontation, action planning and problem solving, team building, inter-group development, evaluation and follow-up.

Organizational behavior model

The organizational behavior model is similar to the organizational development model in that both place importance on the organizations culture. However, organization behavior also studies the individual worker within the organization. People who wish to base their management approach on this model must learn to both understand and predict individual and group behavior, which can be achieved only by evaluating the following four factors: things that occur outside and beyond the control of the organization, the resources that are owned by or accessible to the organization, the past actions of the organization, and form of business strategy. This model is very different from the traditional management of health care organizations.

Nursing model of management

There are three levels to creating a nursing model of management theory, which build upon each other and allow for change once the final stage has been completed. The first step that a nurse manager should be concerned with when forming a personal management model is the foundation. How the individual chooses their foundation depends upon their educational background and professional focus. The following foundations are good examples of where the individual may wish to start: clinical, organizational, and research. The second step in forming a management model is to determine the parts of the system that will be useful to the manager's goals. These things are a few examples of step two: reward systems, percentage of responsibility, communication guidelines and cooperation. The third step in theory development is to review the outcome. These outcomes may be measured by patient satisfaction, staff happiness and patient outcomes. Once all three steps have been completed, the nurse manager can return to step one to make any necessary adjustments.

Stress management

Helping employees learn how to manage stress appropriately is very important in the field of health care. Employees under stress make more errors and in medical organizations, errors can literally cost lives. Nurse administrators should be aware that there are several things that cause stress in the work environment: problems with the amount of work, fast changes, not feeling secure in the job position, having little or no control over decisions that directly affect the work, and bad managers. Stress management can work by preventing stress and teaching ways to deal with stress when it does occur. One of the best and easiest ways to relieve employee stress is to let them know that as a manager you are always available to hear their ideas and complaints.

Drug abuse or theft issues

An often hidden problem in the field of nursing is the theft and/or use of narcotic drugs by nurses. Nurses may also enter the workplace while using other chemical substances such as alcohol. It is very important for managers to be aware of the signs and symptoms related to chemical dependency because it often leads to impairment of practice and medical errors. The following are things to keep a look out for if one suspects a nurse of using drugs: an increase in being late, absent, or using sick time with ambiguous explanations, frequent and long break periods; work becomes inconsistent; record keeping becomes sloppy, often including errors; failure to keep records; and dramatic shifts in mood. Physical signs of drug abuse include hand tremors, restlessness and nausea. Theft of medication can be more difficult to spot but here are some things to watch for: patients supposedly receive more pain medication than average but complain about lack of pain relief, reports of lost or wasted medicine, and offering to work on units that administer large amounts of pain medication.

There are several things a health care organization and nurse managers can do to limit this problem. First, the organization must develop a policy regarding chemical dependency and theft. Second, all staff and personnel should be familiar with the policy. Next, nurses must know that their identity will be kept hidden if they inform a manager about a problem. Once the nurse manager learns of a problem, she should write out a plan of action. The nurse manager needs to keep notes and gather evidence. Then, as quickly as possible, the nurse should be evaluated and if necessary placed on temporary suspension pending a fair hearing. Finally, nurses should be given a choice of treatment options and a way to re-enter the field once they are free from addiction.

Absenteeism

There are two different types of absenteeism that must be addressed in the workplace. Innocent absenteeism refers to workers who do not come to work for reasons that are beyond their control and cannot be dealt with using disciplinary actions. Several steps are used to deal with innocent absenteeism. First, counsel the individual as to the organization's policies on sick leave. If the employee is gone from work only from time to time, meet with them each time they come back to work. If the employee is out for a long time, then call them regularly for updates. If the employee continues to miss a lot of work, give them a written notice of counseling. Next, consider changing the employee's work hours or job description. Finally, work with an arbitrator to consider firing the employee. Culpable absenteeism occurs when the employee willfully misses work. These employees should first be given a verbal then written warning. Next, they should be placed on suspension. Finally, they should be fired.

Change

Kurt Lewin was a social scientist who believed that change occurs only when the status quo is disturbed. He was a proponent of "force field theory": the idea that equilibrium can occur even when some members want change. Lewin defined three steps of change: deciding to change, changing, returning to a state of equilibrium. Lippitt used Lewin's force field theory to form his own seven step model for change. First, the group must decide what the problem is. Second, the ability and will to change must be measured. Third, group members should learn why they want to change and what they will need to create the change. Next, a plan to change one step at a time is created. Then, individuals are given specific roles to play in the facilitation of the change. Once change has occurred, it needs to be evaluated and maintained. Finally, the individuals facilitating the change revert to their normal roles.

In order to keep up with advancing health care, an organization must make frequent changes. The problem is change costs money. For change to occur systems must be analyzed, plans must be created and implemented, and reviews must be undertaken. Over planning and under planning are two of the most costly mistakes an organization can make when attempting to make changes. Over planning happens when management sinks resources into the process of change without first consulting or analyzing staff opinions. Management may have a complete, excellent plan in hand, only for it to be rejected outright or sabotaged by sloppy implementation from staff. Under planning happens when the organization does not think through each step of a change carefully enough. Perhaps they forget to consult local planning commissioners before beginning a construction project or do not consider a project manager necessary to implementation. Whatever the cause, under planning can make an organization halt mid-way, losing the money already invested in the change.

Change theory

There are three main ways that an administrator may bring about change in an organization. If an administrator feels that their employees function rationally in regards to their self-interests then an empirical-rational model is a good way to bring about change. The elements for change using the empirical-rational model must be found researching the organization using the scientific method. This model is particularly helpful when new ideas are needed for the hiring of new staff and keeping current staff on the job. At times, the way in which organizations solve difficulties is in itself the problem, and the normative-reductive method of change can be helpful in solving this dilemma. This method states that people work in order to satisfy their needs. The final category for effecting change is the power-coercive method. At times workers may feel that they are unable to control their own fate and may use the non-violent tactics, striking for example, the power-coercive method in order to effect change.

Diffusion of innovation theory

Much research has been done in order to learn why certain people are better at bringing about change than others. Rogers developed a five step plan to describe how the personality of an individual along with working environment interacts to successfully disperse innovation. First, an individual must learn of a new idea and come to an understanding of why and how it works. Then, the person decides if they like the idea or not. Next, they decide to use the new idea or pass it by and look for something else. Once the innovation has been chosen then it must be put to use. Finally, the decision maker looks to see if the new idea is working. If it is not working then they may scrap it or change it to better fit their needs. IN order for a new innovation or an idea to take hold, the individual must play an active role in implementing and following through with it.

Real-time strategic change

One of the most recent models for bringing about change in an organization was developed by Jacobs in 1994. Jacobs outlines a theory for real-time strategic change. In this theory, all employees, not just managers or facilitators, must take an active role in deciding how to change and then changing together. These steps should occur as one fluid movement rather than in delineated stages, perhaps even as quickly as in one meeting. Jacobs was driven by the idea that because technology is changing so rapidly it is foolish to try to make decisions about change in long drawn out stages. He also insists that other models of change lead to unhappy employees and stagnation as the group will be unable to keep up with the constantly changing outside world.

Management by objectives

Management by objectives (MBO) is the process of helping employees make personal work goals that mirror the organization's goals. The manager should only assess the final performance and not the methods used by the employee to get there. It is important that all employees work on the foundation of organizational goals so that they will completely understand the goals that they must reach. The acronym SMART is used to determine whether objectives have been set properly. "S" stands for specific; because objectives should be outlined as completely as possible. Goals must also be "measurable" so that the employee and management can track progress. The limitations of both employee and organization are remembered with "A" achievable and "R" realistic. Finally, objective should be based on a "time" limit.

Mentoring

Developing and maintaining a mentoring program has many positive outcomes for health care organizations and individuals. More experienced nurses work with those less experienced or new to the facility. Mentoring gives both participants a solid framework to base an ongoing collaborative relationship. Nurses with mentors are more likely to stay on the job and less likely to make errors. Also, nurses with mentors go further in their careers than those who do not have mentors. The following are some of the characteristics of a good mentor: shows through their actions how to be professional, helps the one being mentored to make connections with other colleagues, offers to listen to problems, helps the nurse to make goals and solve problems, expects the best, improves self-confidence.

Practice Test

Practice Questions

1. Fogging is a communication technique for managing criticism, which allows a person to:
   a. agree in principle and receive criticism without becoming defensive.
   b. encourage others to communicate assertively.
   c. use distraction to avoid acknowledgment of the criticism.
   d. use intimidation to redirect the conversation.

2. A nurse executive is most likely use which of the following decision-making models to implement a nursing program that requires evaluation after implementation?
   a. Bureaucratic Model
   b. Collegial Model
   c. Cybernetic Model
   d. Garbage Can Model

3. All of the following questions would be considered acceptable to ask a prospective employee during an interview EXCEPT:
   a. have you worked for this hospital in the past under a different name?
   b. do you feel you will be able to perform the duties of this position?
   c. are you authorized to work in the United States?
   d. how many children do you have?

4. Nursing staff in an emergency department labeled a patient as "borderline," "attention seeker," and a "services abuser." Nursing documentation in the patient's record reflects these views, including additional statements, such as the patient "shows up at least once a week with various complaints." On one visit, the patient complained of abdominal pain and vomiting. Minimal treatment was provided, and the patient was discharged. Later, the staff is informed that the patient required surgery at another hospital for an intestinal blockage; litigation is pending. The defense attorneys reviewed all existing nursing documentation. It is likely that the nursing staff in the Emergency Department will be charged with:
   a. slander
   b. libel.
   c. harassment.
   d. unintentional tort.

5. In all 50 states, minors can provide informed consent for:
   a. HIV testing and treatment.
   b. sexually transmitted disease testing and treatment except for HIV.
   c. contraceptive services.
   d. abortion.

6. Paternalistic actions are incompatible with nursing ethics because they:
   a. reduce ethical obligation.
   b. reduce the accountability of the nurse.
   c. decrease the authority of the nurse.
   d. diminish the autonomy of the patient.

7. The nursing care delivery model in which a nurse holds 24-hour responsibility for a patient from admission through discharge is known as:
   a. team nursing.
   b. modular nursing
   c. functional nursing.
   d. primary nursing.

8. A patient classification system is used to measure:
   a. customer satisfaction.
   b. acuity level.
   c. performance variations.
   d. patient safety.

9. The original purpose for the development of diagnosis-related groups was to:
   a. determine Medicare reimbursement at a fixed-fee.
   b. provide funding for private insurance companies.
   c. determine prescription drug benefits.
   d. provide sliding-scale reimbursement for Medicare beneficiaries.

10. Medical waste disposal programs are primarily regulated at the:
   a. federal level.
   b. local level.
   c. state level.
   d. community level.

11. The Patient Self-Determination Act requires federally funded hospitals to provide:
   a. written notice to patients regarding their rights to make treatment decisions.
   b. treatment to patients who are uninsured.
   c. reasonable accommodation to patients with disabilities.
   d. protection to patients by making nurses accountable through practice regulations.

12. The business analysis technique most likely to be used by a nurse executive for strategic planning is known as:
   a. VPEC-T analysis.
   b. SWOT analysis.
   c. MoSCow analysis.
   d. PC analysis.

13. The budget method that requires a comprehensive review and justification of all expenditures before resources are allocated is known as:
    a. incremental budgeting.
    b. priority-based budgeting.
    c. activity-based budgeting.
    d. zero-based budgeting.

14. Fifty new hospital beds are required to replace beds with faulty rails on several units. The funds for these new beds are allocated from which type of budget?
    a. Capital budget
    b. Operational budget
    c. Labor budget
    d. Marketing budget

15. A comparison of hospital services to the best practices of other industries with similar services with the goal of establishing higher standards is one example of:
    a. networking.
    b. market research.
    c. quantitative research.
    d. benchmarking.

16. Which component of the nursing process may be delegated with supervision?
    a. Assessment
    b. Planning
    c. Intervention
    d. Evaluation

17. Standards of the Occupational Safety and Health Administration require that all new employees who provide direct care must:
    a. be offered the hepatitis B three-injection series vaccination.
    b. have an annual TB test.
    c. accept evaluation by a health care provider in the event of a needle stick.
    d. obtain a titer following hepatitis B three-injection series vaccination.

18. Which of the following laws was passed in 2002 to address the nursing shortage through retention and recruitment initiatives?
    a. Model Nursing Practice Act
    b. America's Partnership for Nursing Education Act
    c. National Nurse Act
    d. Nurse Reinvestment Act

19. Which of the following statements regarding the privacy rules of the Health Insurance Portability and Accountability Act (HIPAA) is correct?
   a. HIPAA privacy rules authorize covered entities to disclose protected health information without an individual's authorization in the event of a public health emergency.
   b. HIPAA privacy rules authorize covered entities to impose fees for searching and retrieving copies of medical records when copies of records are requested.
   c. HIPAA privacy rules authorize covered entities to retain tape-recorded information, following transcription of medical information.
   d. HIPAA privacy rules restrict an individual's access to their medical record, following a clinical trial.

20. Which quantitative research methodology focuses on the statistical analysis of multiple research studies on a selected topic with the goal of investigating study characteristics and integrating the results?
   a. Meta-analysis
   b. Survey
   c. Needs assessment
   d. Methodological study

21. Federal regulation regarding Institutional Review Boards has which of the following characteristics?
   a. They may consist entirely of members from the same profession.
   b. They should not include a member whose primary concerns are nonscientific.
   c. They may invite experts in special areas to vote on complex issues.
   d. They must include one member who is not affiliated with the institution.

22. Health care organizations may categorize customers as external or internal. An example of an external customer is:
   a. a hospital-based physician.
   b. a contracted managed care company.
   c. patient care staff.
   d. a hospital administrator.

23. Recently, the nursing staff has been notified that their medical surgical unit will be relocated to another building on campus to allow for the construction of a new intensive care unit. Several of the nurses are complaining about moving to a smaller unit and are verbalizing possibilities of decreases in staffing and compromised patient care. An effective change agent should do which of the following?
   a. Hold a department meeting to notify nursing staff that the move is mandatory and not debatable.
   b. Recommend that staff nurses prepare a formal written complaint, which will be presented to administration.
   c. Avoid acknowledgment of complaints, and move forward to discourage additional negative communication.
   d. Involve staff nurses in the move, including staff meetings to provide information and receive feedback.

24. Which of the following conflict resolution styles includes both parties actively attempting to find solutions that will satisfy goals of both parties?
   a. Avoidance
   b. Accommodation
   c. Compromise
   d. Collaboration

25. Under the Fair Labor Standards Act, which of the following statements concerns exempt employees?
   a. They must be paid for 7 holidays a year if working 40 hours a week.
   b. They must be paid overtime if they work more than a 40-hour week.
   c. They are salaried employees and are not subject to minimum wage.
   d. They must receive a minimum of one break period for each 4 hours of work.

26. Expectations of the Joint Commission's Sentinel Event Policy for accredited hospitals include all the following EXCEPT to:
   a. report all defined sentinel events.
   b. B. conduct a root-cause analysis within 45 days of becoming aware of a reviewable sentinel event.
   c. define all events within the hospital that are subject to review under the Sentinel
   d. Event Policy.
   e. develop an action plan and respond appropriately to defined sentinel events.

27. Which of the following is an example of a reviewable sentinel event as defined by the Joint Commission's Sentinel Event Policy?
   a. Patient death, following a discharge "against medical advice"
   b. Unsuccessful suicide attempt without major loss of permanent function
   c. Employee death, following blood-borne pathogen exposure
   d. Patient fall, resulting in permanent loss of function

28. As part of the Joint Commission's National Patient Safety Goal, a list of "do not use" abbreviations, acronyms, and symbols was developed for accredited hospitals to assist in attaining the safety goal. Which of the following is a "do not use" value symbol in medication orders?
   a. 1.0 mg
   b. 1 mg
   c. 0.1 mg
   d. 1 mL

29. For a nurse to be held liable for malpractice, all of the following elements must be proved EXCEPT that:
   a. a nurse–patient relationship existed.
   b. standards of care were breached by the nurse.
   c. injury or damage was suffered by the patient.
   d. there was a direct cause between the nurse's actions and the patient's injury.

30. The Health Insurance Portability and Accountability Act (HIPAA) privacy rule allows the disclosure of protected health information for clinical research under all of the following circumstances EXCEPT:
   a. the subject has signed valid Privacy Rule Authorization.
   b. a waiver was granted by an Institutional Review Board or Privacy Board.
   c. protected health information has been de-identified.
   d. the subject has signed an informed consent.

31. Under the Health Insurance Portability and Accountability Act (HIPAA) Privacy Rule, protected health information may be disclosed following de-identification. Which of the following descriptive elements of an individual would not require removal during the de-identifying process?
   a. Date of birth
   b. State
   c. Social security number
   d. Electronic mail addresses

32. The five-stage model called Tuckman's stages, regarding group dynamics, is often used in decision-making groups. In which of the following stages would a leader clarify roles and rules for working collaboratively and team members begin to build a commitment to the team goal?
   a. Norming
   b. Storming
   c. Performing
   d. Forming

33. In which of the following types of leadership power do followers comply, not for rewards or the possibility of negative consequences, but because the leader is perceived to have the authority to direct others?
   a. Referent power
   b. Legitimate power
   c. Expert power
   d. Coercive power

34. A newly licensed nurse accepted a position on a medical unit. As part of the orientation process, he was assigned a preceptor for 4 weeks. Over time, the nurse noticed that his preceptor consistently provided only partial answers to many important questions, often in a condescending tone, and frequently stated "You do not need to know that right now." This type of behavior is known as:
   a. clinical violence.
   b. verbal abuse.
   c. intimidation.
   d. lateral violence.

35. A standard Centers for Disease Control case form must be completed for which of the following notifiable infectious diseases?
   a. Campylobacteriosis
   b. Listeriosis
   c. Histoplasmosis
   d. Leptospirosis

36. The Department of Health and Human Services division responsible for investigating Medicare fraud is the office of:
   a. Medicare Hearings and Appeals.
   b. Global Health Affairs.
   c. Inspector General.
   d. Intergovernmental Affairs.

37. The American Nurses Association Principals for Nurse Staffing questions the usefulness of which the following factors when determining staffing plans?
   a. Nursing hours per patient day
   b. Number of patients
   c. Available technology
   d. Staff experience and skill level

38. An example of centralized decision-making is:
   a. staff members participate in self-scheduling.
   b. the nurse manager approves all new hires through the nurse executive.
   c. nurses provide care based on the Primary Nursing Model.
   d. a committee of nurses is formed to engage in quality-improvement initiatives.

39. A unit manager notifies the nurse executive of her intent to resign because she is unable meet the recently reduced expectations for staff budgeting. The cognitive distortion of the nurse manager is known as:
   a. fortune telling.
   b. disqualifying the positive.
   c. catastrophizing.
   d. all-or-nothing thinking.

40. Which of the following statements best describes the Belmont Report?
   a. It makes specific recommendations for Health and Human Services (HHS) administrative action, regarding unethical treatment of human subjects in research.
   b. It defines regulations for human subject protection during research.
   c. It is based on the ethical principles of justice, autonomy, and respect.
   d. It identifies ethical principles, which form the basis of the HHS human subject protection regulations.

41. The U.S. Equal Employment Opportunity Commission (EEOC) enforces federal laws against discrimination in the workplace. Which of the following statements best describes what is least likely to be prohibited by the EEOC employment laws and regulations?
   a. Advertising for employment, seeking female staff only
   b. Recruiting by word-of-mouth, resulting in an almost entirely similar workforce
   c. Reducing benefits for older workers if the reduction results in matching the cost benefits to younger workers
   d. Requesting a photograph of an applicant during the initial hiring process

42. The overall goal of Healthy People 2020 is to:
   a. promote health and prevent disease for all Americans.
   b. track national disease data over 10 years.
   c. educate public health workers on leading causes of disease.
   d. compile evidence-based literature on public health issues.

43. What type of insurance covers employers against litigation as a result of negligence by employees for work-related accidents?
   a. Workers' Compensation Insurance
   b. Employer's Liability Insurance
   c. Public Liability Insurance
   d. Keyman Insurance

44. What part of the Medicare program provides optional private health insurance?
   a. Part A
   b. Part B
   c. Part C
   d. Part D

45. What condition is no longer covered by Medicare under the Deficit Reduction Act?
   a. Urinary tract infection
   b. Blood administration
   c. Bypass surgery
   d. Air embolism

46. To comply with the Occupational Safety and Health Administration requirements for an Exposure Control Plan, all of the following elements must be included in the plan EXCEPT:
   a. an exposure determination, identifying job classifications.
   b. procedures to evaluate exposure events.
   c. implementation of methods of exposure control.
   d. a list of all hazardous chemicals and material safety data sheets.

47. Which of the following quality-improvement methods is used to identify and prevent potential problems?
   a. Root-cause analysis
   b. Barrier analysis
   c. Causal factor analysis
   d. Failure mode and effects analysis

48. Which analysis tool is based on the 80/20 rule (80% of problems are caused by 20% of the causes)?
    a. Pareto chart
    b. Run chart
    c. Gantt chart
    d. Flow chart

49. What is the difference between a Gantt chart and the Program Evaluation Review Technique (PERT) chart?
    a. Dependencies between activities in Gantt charts are easier to follow than PERT charts.
    b. Gantt charts are usually preferable to PERT charts for large projects.
    c. Activity times are represented by arrows between activity nodes in Gantt charts.
    d. PERT is a flow chart, and Gantt is a bar chart.

50. What nonprofit organization accredits health plans, individual physicians, and medical groups and provides additional programs, such as credential verification and a multicultural health care distinction?
    a. Joint Commission
    b. National Nonprofit Accreditation Center
    c. Council on Accreditation
    d. National Committee for Quality Assurance

51. According to Healthy People 2020, what is the most preventable cause of disease and death in the United States?
    a. Obesity
    b. Tobacco use
    c. Sexually transmitted diseases
    d. Poor diet and low physical activity

Answer Key and Explanations

1. A: Communication skills are required to develop professional relationships. Assertive communication incorporates sincerity, timing, gestures, and content. Fogging is a communication technique that allows a manager to remain sincere by agreeing in principle without becoming defensive. This passive skill allows the manager to maintain control over the direction of the conversation and discourages the critic from becoming more assertive. As with all communication skills, to be successful, this technique must be selected for the appropriate situation and would not be indicated with aggressive criticism.

2. C: The Cybernetic Model may be used by nurse executives who wish to implement programs that require evaluation. The Cybernetic Model includes three phases: Needs Assessment, Program Implementation, and Results Assessment. In phase 3, program objectives, cost, and impact are evaluated. The Collegial Model involves the collaboration and consensus of a group of peers and is often used in educational settings where professions share similar values and benefit from individual expertise. The Collegial Model approach to decision-making is suited for small-size groups. The Bureaucratic Model is used within a hierarchical organization, such as health care organizations, where operational policies and procedures are used to make decisions. While efficient implementation is gained with this model, creativity and process improvement may be diminished as a result of adherence to governing operations. The Garbage Can Model is based on accidental decision-making where changes may be implemented without a clear plan or actual problem identification.

3. D: Although the interviewer should be in control during the interview process, certain questions are not acceptable. To ask if an interviewee has children or is planning to have children may result in legal proceedings. If the rationale is to assess availability, inquiring about the number of hours the interviewee is available each week is prudent. Questions directly relating to nationality, native language, age, gender, race, disability, place of birth, and marital or family status are discriminatory. The interviewer's goal should be to choose the best candidate for the position in the presence of nondiscriminatory policies. Questions should relate to the position being offered and not to personal information.

4. B: Defamation of character is a type of intentional tort and refers to the communication of ideas that result in a negative image. The two types of defamation of character are slander and libel. Slander refers to spoken words as compared to libel, which refers to written words. Importantly, it is not always necessary that slander or libel be false information. In the scenario described in the question, even if the patient had a diagnosis of borderline personality disorder, when staff documented that the patient was "a borderline," it was not intended to benefit the patient and may, in fact, reduced the patient's chances of receiving adequate treatment. Nurses must remember to identify correctly the purpose of documentation. Nursing documentation must not hinder treatment or cause damage to the patient.

5. B: All 50 states allow minors to consent to sexually transmitted disease testing and treatment except for HIV. Approximately 26 states have passed laws allowing minors to

consent to contraceptive services. State laws vary widely regarding the ability of a minor to provide informed consent for HIV testing and treatment. Very few states allow minors to consent to abortion. It is particularly important to remember that informed consent for a procedure or treatment for any minor or adult may not be provided by a registered nurse. Only the primary provider, such as a physician or nurse practitioner, may provide the information required for informed consent.

6. D: Paternalistic actions and attitudes diminish the patient's autonomy. Paternalism relates to using one's own judgment to make decisions for another without considering their ideas. In this context, the principles of autonomy and beneficence are in conflict and create an ethical challenge. While respect for the autonomy of the patient should be observed, nurses and other health care providers must implement sound judgment under the principle of beneficence. To meet this challenge, nurses must recognize the importance of personal choice and equality in a professional nurse–patient relationship.

7. D: The framework of how nursing care is delivered in an organization is called a nursing care delivery model. There are four classic models; total patient care, functional nursing, team nursing, and primary nursing. In the total patient care model, a patient receives complete care by one nurse for an entire shift. In a functional nursing model, tasks are divided for groups of patients. The registered nurse (RN) performs advanced nursing functions for a group of patients, and other tasks, such as personal care and vital signs, may be assigned to ancillary staff members. In team nursing, an RN team leader manages care for a small group of patients by planning and delegating tasks to team members. Primary nursing is different from the total patient care model in that the RN holds 24-hour responsibility for the communication and direction of each patient's care, although some patient care may be delegated to support staff.

8. B: Nurse executives play a key role in the development of effective patient classification systems (PCS). A PCS is used to measure the level and amount of care or the acuity level for specific populations of patients. Examples include medical, pediatric, ambulatory, and psychiatric classification systems. One of the main goals in the development of a PCS is ensuring the delivery of safe care by providing appropriate staffing levels with competent personnel to care for patients from a specific population. Other goals include maintaining customer and staff satisfaction while adhering to financial resources.

9. A: In 1983, the Social Security Act was amended to include a prospective payment system for Medicare beneficiaries. Diagnosis-related groups (DRGs) were originally designed as part of a classification system used by Medicare to determine reimbursement at a fixed-fee. DRGs are based on several factors, including the International Classification of Disease diagnoses, procedures, age, and the presence of comorbidities. Since the amendment, health care has evolved, leading to specialized types of DRGs, such as All Patient DRGs and Refined DRGs.

10. A: The Environmental Protection Agency (EPA) implements laws by writing regulations and setting national standards that protect human health and the environment. The EPA regulates hazardous waste at the federal level and provides model guidelines for state medical waste management programs. Biomedical waste programs and disposal are primarily regulated at the state level. Laws vary depending on state. The web site, www.epa.gov, can be visited for additional information.

11. A: The Patient Self-Determination Act (PSDA), a federal statute, was an amendment to the Omnibus Budget Reconciliation Act of 1990. The PSDA requires federally funded health care facilities, such as hospitals, hospice providers, and nursing homes, to provide information in writing regarding advanced health care directives on admission. The purpose of the PSDA is to ensure that patients are aware of their right to make treatment decisions and that these decisions are communicated to their health care provider. On admission, patients must be asked if they have a living will or a durable power of attorney, and responses should be documented in the patient's medical record.

12. B: A SWOT analysis would most likely be used in strategic planning. SWOT analyses focus on the objective assessment of four main attributes: strengths, weaknesses, opportunities, and threats; these analyses are useful in developing strategic responses to opportunities and challenges. A VPEC-T analysis is often used to analyze expectations of involved parties without losing information in the transition from business needs to information technology development. The MoSCow analysis is also a business technique used in software development. The PC analysis, or principal component analysis, is a statistical tool used for multivariate analyses.

13. D: The zero-based budgeting method requires that all expenditures be justified for each new period (starting at a zero base). This budget method is time-consuming but provides more accurate and current results. Incremental budgeting is based on the previous budget and incorporates adjustments for additional planned increases, such as inflation and salary raises. Priority-based budgeting involves the development of a prioritization plan when determining the allocation of resources. The activity-based budgeting method focuses on creating a budget based on costs of key activities and their relationship to strategic goals.

14. A: A capital budget is developed to purchase long-term assets, such as equipment, computer hardware, and building facilities. It may require several years to pay off these assets, and they are called capital assets because of their multiyear value. The operational budget represents the total value of all resources and expenses of a department or organization. Additional budgets, such as a labor budget, are subcategories of the operational budget.

15. D: There are several types of benchmarking, including generic, global, performance, and functional benchmarking. Additionally, benchmarking may occur at different levels, such as the best in an industry, internal or competitive. For example, internal benchmarking may occur in a hospital where each department's check out services are compared and evaluated to determine the best internal practices. These best practices are then implemented across all hospital departments.

16. C: When registered nurses (RNs) delegate tasks, they remain accountable for the overall care of the patient. Therefore, RNs must be aware of the qualifications of assistive personnel to delegate tasks appropriately. The American Nurses Association (ANA) provides guidelines and principles on delegation in the document "ANA Principles for Delegation." In addition to the ANA guidelines, delegation is addressed specifically by each state nursing practice act. Interventions may be delegated unless they require professional nursing judgment, knowledge, and skill to be completed. For example, the administration of oral medication for a stable patient may be delegated, but an initial nursing assessment may not be delegated.

17. A: Federal standards of the Occupational Safety and Health Administration (OSHA) require that new employees with the potential to be exposed to blood-borne pathogens be offered the hepatitis B three-injection series vaccination within 10 days of employment. New employees have the right to decline the vaccination, which should be documented in the employee's health file. A Hepatitis B Vaccine Declination is mandatory per OSHA standard 1910.1030 App A. OSHA does not require employees working in a health care environment to have an annual tuberculosis (TB) test; the Centers for Disease Control provides guidelines regarding TB testing, which have been adapted by many state regulations. Regarding postexposure evaluation and treatment of a needle stick, OSHA standards require that the employer offer evaluation at no cost; however, an employee may decline. All postexposure treatment accepted or declined, should be documented in the employee's health file. OSHA standards do not require employees to have a titer following hepatitis B three-injection series vaccination. OSHA reports that every year, approximately 8700 health care workers are infected with hepatitis B, resulting in about 200 deaths a year.

18. D: The Nurse Reinvestment Act was passed in 2002 with the support of the American Nurses Association. The Act addresses the nursing shortage by authorizing several provisions, including loan repayment programs, long-term care training grants, and public service announcements to encourage people to enter the nursing profession. The Model Nursing Practice Act, developed by the National Council of State Boards of Nursing, was designed to provide guidelines for State Nurse Practice Acts. America's Partnership for Nursing Education Act of 2009 is currently a bill requesting an amendment to the Public Health Service Act. This amendment would make grants available to states with increasing population growth and a projected nursing shortage. The grants would be used to increase nursing faculty in those states. The National Nurse Act is another bill that was introduced in the House of Representatives on February 4, 2010. The bill is an amendment to establish the Office of the National Nurse with the same rank and grade as the Deputy Surgeon General of the Public Health Services. Duties of the National Nurse would include, but are not limited to, guidance and leadership in encouraging nurses to become nurse educators and increasing public safety and emergency preparedness.

19. A: Health care providers may share protected information to prevent or decrease an imminent threat to the public. The Health Insurance Portability and Accountability Act (HIPAA) privacy rules permit covered entities to impose reasonable fees for copying and mailing requested medical records. However, the fee may not include costs for searching or retrieving the requested information. HIPAA privacy rules do not require covered entities to retain tape-recorded information, following transcription of medical information. HIPAA rules permit temporary restrictions on individual access to medical information if involved in a clinical trial, providing the participant agreed during initial consent. However, the researcher must inform the participant that access will be reinstated following the clinical trial.

20. A: Meta-analysis is a statistical procedure to integrate the results of several studies on a particular topic. Advantages of meta-analysis include the ability to identify patterns across studies, detecting relationships that may not be identifiable in a single study and greater statistical power. Survey research involves the use of questionnaires or interviews to gather information. Market research, opinion polls, and the census are types of surveys. Surveys are generally less expensive than other types of research, and data collection through the Internet has increased access to larger groups of specific populations. Needs assessment

research focuses on collecting information to determine the needs for a specific group or organization.

21. D: Institutional Review Boards (IRBs) are regulated by the Food and Drug Administration and the Department of Health and Human Services. IRBs are required for all institutions performing research that receive federal funding. The main purpose of an IRB is to protect the rights of research participants. The Code of Federal Regulations contains specific laws regarding IRB membership. No IRB may consist entirely of members of one profession, and each IRB should contain at least one member not affiliated with the institution. Additionally, IRBs should contain at least one member whose primary concerns are in scientific areas and one member whose primary concerns are in nonscientific areas. While an IRB may invite special experts to assist in the review of complex issues, those individuals may not vote with the IRB.

22. B: Health care organizations are unique in that they provide services to many parties including their own suppliers. To help distinguish types of customers, internal customers are identified as individuals or departments working within the hospital who use the hospital's services. Examples of internal customers include patient care staff, hospital-based physicians, and a hospital administrator. External customers are customers who receive services but are not employed at the hospital. Examples of external customers include referring physicians, patients, patient's families, managed care companies contracting with the hospital, and other business entities, such as third-party payers.

23. D: An effective change agent will recognize the importance of sharing goals with staff. Effective change strategies include encouraging involvement by all individuals who will be affected by change and supporting open communication. Additional change strategies include providing education or training if needed to reduce fear and prepare staff to move forward.

24. D: Effectively managed conflict can be beneficial for an organization. Conflict behavior styles include avoidance, accommodation, force, compromise, and collaboration. An awareness of these styles during periods of conflict is useful in determining communication techniques to manage conflict effectively. The avoidance style is nonconfrontational but does not often lead to conflict resolution or goal achievement. When the force style is used, it is considered a win/lose situation, with the opposing goals or values being disregarded. Persons using the accommodating style are nonassertive and cooperative at the expense of their own goals to satisfy others. The collaboration style includes an element of mutual respect where both conflict parties attempt to reach solutions that will retain the goals of both parties. Giving up some aspects of goals through assertive and cooperative behavior is a compromising style. A compromising style results in the partial satisfaction of both parties.

25. C: The Fair Labor Standards Act (FLSA) is a federal law administered by the Department of Labor. The FLSA establishes laws, such as child labor standards, overtime pay, and minimum wage. Employees are classified by the duties and responsibilities associated with their position. Although there are grey areas, nonexempt employees generally hold routine work, are paid hourly, and are entitled to receiving overtime. Exempt employees are exempt from receiving overtime pay and are known as salaried employees. The FLSA does not require payment for time not worked, including vacations or sick time. Additionally, the

FLSA does not require breaks or meal periods to be provided to employees. However, employers must also adhere to additional state labor laws, which may be more detailed regarding breaks and vary from state to state. Some states such as Kentucky, Colorado, and Nevada require a 10-minute break for every 4 hours worked. Florida has no state law regulating rest periods for adult workers.

26. A: The Sentinel Event Policy has four main goals; to improve patient care, reduce the number of sentinel events, increase knowledge regarding sentinel events, and to uphold public confidence in accredited organizations. Although accredited hospitals must define sentinel events within their organization, hospitals are not required to report sentinel events to the Joint Commission. However, if the Joint Commission becomes aware of a reviewable sentinel event through voluntary self-reporting or otherwise, the organization is expected to conduct a root-cause analysis and action plan within 45 days of becoming aware of the sentinel event.

27. D: The Joint Commission Sentinel Event Policy defines both reviewable and nonreviewable sentinel events. Reviewable sentinel events are events that have resulted in unanticipated death or permanent loss of function to patients or residents. Reviewable sentinel events are subject to review by the Joint Commission. Nonreviewable sentinel events include "near miss" incidents, events that have not affected a recipient of care, and deaths or loss of function following an "against medical advice" discharge. For more information on the Joint Commission and the Sentinel Event Policy visit www.jointcommission.org.

28. A: The Joint Commission's official "Do Not Use" List identifies the documentation of trailing zeros (1.0) or lack or a leading zero (.1 mg) to be a potential problem. A missed decimal point may lead to an incorrect interpretation. For example, 1.0 mg may appear as 10 mg if the decimal point was not identified in a physician's order. Similarly .1 mg may appear as 1 mg since it is lacking a leading zero. There is an exception for trailing zeros when reporting necessary increased levels of precision. Laboratory values, imaging studies, and lesion measurements may require trailing zeros for increased precision reporting. Trailing zeros may not be used in medication orders.

29. D: The Joint Commission defines malpractice as improper or unethical conduct or unreasonable lack of skill by a holder of a professional or official position and defines negligence as the failure to use such care as a reasonably prudent and careful person would use under similar circumstances. Several elements must be proven to hold a nurse liable for malpractice. Proof of a causal relationship must be established between the patient's injury and the nurse's failure to adhere to standards of care. However, the relationship must only demonstrate substantial cause.

30. D: The Privacy Rule was issued in 2003 by the U.S. Department of Health and Human Services (DHHS) following the Health Insurance Portability and Accountability Act of 1996. The privacy rule has several effects on clinical research. Personal Health Information (PHI) must be protected during the disclosure of research. A Privacy Rule Authorization must adhere to section 164.508 as outlined in the privacy rule. Core elements of the Privacy Rule Authorization include a description of the protected health information (PHI) to be disclosed, the purpose of the disclosure, an expiration date or notice of no expiration, and a dated signature. In contrast, a signed informed consent is not used for the authorization for

the disclosure of PHI. An informed consent is required by the DHHS and the Food and Drug Administration Protection of Human Subjects Regulations to consent to participate in the research. De-identification of PHI and waivers through an Institutional Review Board or Privacy Board are other possible methods of disclosing certain PHI.

31. B: The de-identifying of information is one method that allows the disclosure of protected health information (PHI) under the Health Insurance Portability and Accountability Act privacy rule for research purposes. There are 18 descriptive elements that must be removed before disclosure to prevent the identification of an individual. Names, geographic subdivisions smaller than a state, element of dates, and any unique identifying numbers, including an electronic mail address and Internet protocol address number are a few of the 18 elements that must be removed during the de-identification of PHI.

32. A: To assist team leaders in accomplishing goals, it is important to understand group dynamics in organizational development. Tuckman's stages initially comprised a four-stage model and later expanded to include a final adjourning stage. In the first stage, called the forming stage, the group forms and initial communication begins. The group leader focuses on communicating the goals of the group. During the second stage, storming, team members may challenge authority and compete for roles. The group leader should facilitate open professional communication, support all members and continue to communicate goals. In the norming stage, hierarchy has been established, and the team begins to focus on the goals. The group leader promotes a cohesive team atmosphere. In the performing stage, members are working collaboratively toward goals. The final adjourning stage concludes a decision-making group.

33. B: Legitimate power is based upon the leader's position of authority in the organization. Referent power is created when the follower identifies positively with characteristics and qualities of the leader. Expert power is created when followers believe the leader has expert knowledge and competence. Coercive power is based on threat of punishment. Both expert and referent types of power indicate positive attitudes of followers toward their leaders, which enhances respect and commitment rather than simple compliance.

34. D: Lateral violence or horizontal violence between nurses is not uncommon and is often directed toward new nurses. Forms of lateral violence include sabotage, withholding information (as noted in the scenario described in the question), and nonverbal gestures, such as face-making. Managing lateral violence in the health care setting is challenging as this type of violence is frequently covert and met with denial during confrontation. Proactive education and policies regarding zero-tolerance to violence in the workplace can reduce unprofessional behavior. The Joint Commission issued a Sentinel Event Alert in 2008 on behaviors that undermine a culture of safety. The alert includes recommendations for reducing intimidating and disruptive behavior. For more information, the following web site can be visited:
http://www.jointcommission.org/SentinelEvents/SentinelEventAlert/sea_40.htm.

35. B: State and local laws require health care providers and laboratories to report specific infectious diseases to the state or public health authority. The state health department then compiles the data and reports nationally notifiable infectious diseases to the Centers for Disease Control (CDC) through the National Notifiable Diseases Surveillance System

(NNDSS). The list of nationally notifiable infectious diseases is revised as necessary and is available for review on the CDC web site. Morbidity and mortality weekly reports are generated from the data. Listeriosis is an infection caused by the bacteria *Listeria monocytogenes* and has been nationally reportable since 2000. In addition to national reporting, all persons with listeriosis should be interviewed by a health care provider, using the standard CDC *Listeria* case form. Although relatively rare, cases of listeriosis have risen since 2002. There are several methods of transmission, the most common of which is through ingestion of contaminated food, such as undercooked meat or contaminated vegetables, seafood, and dairy products. Direct contact may cause skin lesions. Flu-like symptoms, such as fever and muscle aches, are common with listeriosis infections. However, *Listeria* can infect the brain or spinal cord and may be transferred to a fetus in utero or during birth.

36. C: The mission of the Office of Inspector General (OIG) as mandated by public law includes protecting programs of the Department of Health and Human Services. The OIG, the Federal Bureau of Investigation, and the Department of Justice are federal agencies that collaborate with state agencies to detect and prevent fraud. Medicare and Medicaid fraud may be reported directly to the OIG for investigation. Examples of Medicare fraud include submitting false claims, door-to-door solicitation of beneficiaries, payment for referrals by Medicare providers, and misrepresentation of Medicare private plans.

37. A: In 1998, the American Nurses Association (ANA) developed the Utilization Guide to the Principles on Safe Staffing. Nine principles for safe staffing are identified within three categories; patient care unit–related staffing, staff-related staffing, and institution/organization–related staffing. Patient care unit–related staffing principle s identify critical factors for consideration when determining a staffing plan, which include the number of patients, the level of experience and education of staff, and contextual issues, such as available technology. The guide questions the use of nursing hours per patient days (NHPPDs) in the development of staffing plans. NHPPDs do not reflect the variability of factors necessary to predict the requirements for every possible type of patient care setting. Averaging hours of care for each patient as opposed to measuring the intensity of care required is not appropriate in nursing practice. The Utilization Guide may be accessed at: www.safestaffingsaveslives.org.

38. B: Centralized decision-making occurs when the span of authority and the control of key business elements are retained by top-level management. Decision-making is not disbursed. Two advantages of centralization are the ability to make rapid decisions and consistency in communication. Obvious disadvantages are the possibilities of being managed by a dictator and the loss of employee creativity and knowledge.

39. D: During verbal communication, it is important to actively listen and understand possible cognitive distortions to identify pertinent facts and avoid misunderstandings and conflict. In the scenario described in the question, the nurse executive should recognize that the nurse manager is using all-or-nothing thinking. All-or-nothing, or black and white thinking, is often noted in perfectionists who are unable to meet unreasonable demands. The nurse manager sees herself as a failure because of her inability to complete the task. It would be prudent for the nurse executive to investigate the staff budgeting rather than focus on the manager's competence.

40. D: Published in 1978, the Ethical Principles and Guidelines for the Protection of Human Subjects of Research became known as the Belmont Report. The guidelines identify three ethical principles regarding the use of human subjects in research; respect, beneficence, and justice. These ethical principles are applied directly to research and pertain to informed, voluntary participation and protection of human subjects. Although the Belmont Report does not make specific recommendations or define regulations for human subjects of research, federal regulations under the HHS are based on these guidelines.

41. C: The Equal Employment Opportunity commission (EEOC) enforces federal laws against discrimination as a result of race, color, religion, sex, national origin, age, disability, and genetics. It is illegal to base wages or benefits on the discriminatory factors listed. Reducing benefits for older workers (if the reduction is equal to the cost of benefits for younger workers), may be legal in certain situations. It is important to note that discrimination based on sex also includes pregnant women, and discrimination based on age mainly focuses on persons over 40 years of age.

42. A: Healthy People 2020 (HP2020) is a health promotion and disease prevention program initiated in January 2000 by the United States Department of Health and Human Services. HP2020 consists of 42 categories and hundreds of health goals and objectives. National data from 190 data sources have been gathered over the last 10 years to measure the outcomes for the objectives. Collected data are based on a list of leading health indicators, which include physical activity, obesity, tobacco use, and access to health care, among others. Progress reviews analyze the data based on the 28 focus areas

43. B: Employers' Liability Insurance protects employers against lawsuits of negligence or failure to provide safe working conditions. Many Workers' Compensation policies include a separate section for Employer's Liability coverage. Most states have laws requiring both types of insurance. Employers' Liability coverage does not protect against litigation related to discrimination. Public Liability Insurance provides insurance against third-party injuries.

44. C: Medicare Part C offers Medicare Advantage Plans, and enrolled participants receive all Medicare-covered care through private health insurance. To qualify for enrollment, applicants must have Medicare Part A and Part B. The Centers of Medicaid and Medicare forecast that they will serve over 98 million Americans at a cost of 803.1 billion dollars, not including non-benefit administrative costs for the fiscal year of 2010.

45. D: Under section 5001(c) of the Deficit Reduction Act, the Centers for Medicare and Medicaid no longer cover certain illnesses acquired during hospitalization. The list of illnesses includes pressure ulcers stages III and IV, certain infections following surgery, vascular and urinary catheter infections, air embolisms, administration of incompatible blood, and foreign objects unintentionally retained after surgery.

46. D: An Exposure Control Plan (ECP) should include several elements: determination of employee exposure, implementation of methods of exposure control, hepatitis B vaccination documentation, postexposure evaluation, employee training, recordkeeping, and procedures to evaluate exposure events. Lists of hazardous chemicals and material safety data sheets are also requirements of the Occupational Safety and Health Administration within the Hazardous Communication Program. Templates for an ECP and a Hazardous

Communication Program are available for review at:
http://www.osha.gov/Publications/osha3186.pdf.

47. D: A failure mode and effects analysis (FMEA) is a method used to identify potential failure modes or processes. Possible effects of those failures are analyzed and action recommendations are formulated. Benefits of regularly performing a FMEA include identifying change requirements, preventing negative occurrences, and improving patient care through prevention planning. A root-cause analysis is reactive to adverse occurrences and is performed following an event to investigate root causes.

48. A: The Pareto principle, also known as the 80/20 rule was initially created by Italian economist Vilfredo Pareto. The principle was based on a mathematical formula that was developed to analyze the unequal distribution of wealth in early 1900 Italy. In 1941, Dr. J. Juran, a quality-management consultant identified that Pareto's formula could be applied to other areas beyond economics, namely quality. The Pareto principal quickly became a useful analysis tool in many disciplines. Because of the 80/20 rule, the Pareto chart is useful in focusing and prioritizing significant factors or causes.

49. D: Gantt charts are linear bar charts used to display a project schedule. They are effective for small projects with up to 30 activities. While Gantt charts focus on schedule management and time, PERT flow charts focus on the relationship between activities and are often used for large complex projects because they can display connecting dependent networks of activities better than Gantt charts.

50. D: The National Committee for Quality Assurance (NCQA) is a non-profit organization that promotes quality in health care. NCQA offers several accrediting programs for health plans, managed behavioral health care organizations, medical groups, and physicians. A multicultural health care distinction is available through NCQA. The distinction is available for organizations that meet evidence-based criteria for cultural competency.

51. B: Tobacco use is a leading health indicator for Healthy People 2020 (HP2020). HP2020 reports that cigarette smoking is the most preventable cause of disease and death in the United States, and approximately $50 billion is spent annually in direct medical costs as a result of smoking. HP2020 objectives regarding tobacco use include reducing cigarette smoking by adults and adolescents. The Centers for Disease Control report that cigarette smoking causes 1 of every 5 deaths in the United States each year.

Secret Key #1 - Time is Your Greatest Enemy

Pace Yourself

Wear a watch. At the beginning of the test, check the time (or start a chronometer on your watch to count the minutes), and check the time after every few questions to make sure you are "on schedule."

If you are forced to speed up, do it efficiently. Usually one or more answer choices can be eliminated without too much difficulty. Above all, don't panic. Don't speed up and just begin guessing at random choices. By pacing yourself, and continually monitoring your progress against your watch, you will always know exactly how far ahead or behind you are with your available time. If you find that you are one minute behind on the test, don't skip one question without spending any time on it, just to catch back up. Take 15 fewer seconds on the next four questions, and after four questions you'll have caught back up. Once you catch back up, you can continue working each problem at your normal pace.

Furthermore, don't dwell on the problems that you were rushed on. If a problem was taking up too much time and you made a hurried guess, it must be difficult. The difficult questions are the ones you are most likely to miss anyway, so it isn't a big loss. It is better to end with more time than you need than to run out of time.

Lastly, sometimes it is beneficial to slow down if you are constantly getting ahead of time. You are always more likely to catch a careless mistake by working more slowly than quickly, and among very high-scoring test takers (those who are likely to have lots of time left over), careless errors affect the score more than mastery of material.

Secret Key #2 - Guessing is not Guesswork

You probably know that guessing is a good idea - unlike other standardized tests, there is no penalty for getting a wrong answer. Even if you have no idea about a question, you still have a 20-25% chance of getting it right.

Most test takers do not understand the impact that proper guessing can have on their score. Unless you score extremely high, guessing will significantly contribute to your final score.

Monkeys Take the Test

What most test takers don't realize is that to insure that 20-25% chance, you have to guess randomly. If you put 20 monkeys in a room to take this test, assuming they answered once per question and behaved themselves, on average they would get 20-25% of the questions correct. Put 20 test takers in the room, and the average will be much lower among guessed questions. Why?

1. The test writers intentionally write deceptive answer choices that "look" right. A test taker has no idea about a question, so picks the "best looking" answer, which is often wrong. The monkey has no idea what looks good and what doesn't, so will consistently be lucky about 20-25% of the time.

2. Test takers will eliminate answer choices from the guessing pool based on a hunch or intuition. Simple but correct answers often get excluded, leaving a 0% chance of being correct. The monkey has no clue, and often gets lucky with the best choice.

This is why the process of elimination endorsed by most test courses is flawed and detrimental to your performance- test takers don't guess, they make an ignorant stab in the dark that is usually worse than random.

$5 Challenge

Let me introduce one of the most valuable ideas of this course- the $5 challenge:

You only mark your "best guess" if you are willing to bet $5 on it.
You only eliminate choices from guessing if you are willing to bet $5 on it.

Why $5? Five dollars is an amount of money that is small yet not insignificant, and can really add up fast (20 questions could cost you $100). Likewise, each answer choice on one question of the test will have a small impact on your overall score, but it can really add up to a lot of points in the end.

The process of elimination IS valuable. The following shows your chance of guessing it right:

If you eliminate wrong answer choices until only this many remain:	1	2	3
Chance of getting it correct:	100%	50%	33%

However, if you accidentally eliminate the right answer or go on a hunch for an incorrect answer, your chances drop dramatically: to 0%. By guessing among all the answer choices, you are GUARANTEED to have a shot at the right answer.

That's why the $5 test is so valuable- if you give up the advantage and safety of a pure guess, it had better be worth the risk.

What we still haven't covered is how to be sure that whatever guess you make is truly random. Here's the easiest way:

Always pick the first answer choice among those remaining.

Such a technique means that you have decided, **before you see a single test question**, exactly how you are going to guess- and since the order of choices tells you nothing about which one is correct, this guessing technique is perfectly random.

This section is not meant to scare you away from making educated guesses or eliminating choices- you just need to define when a choice is worth eliminating. The $5 test, along with a pre-defined random guessing strategy, is the best way to make sure you reap all of the benefits of guessing.

Secret Key #3 - Practice Smarter, Not Harder

Many test takers delay the test preparation process because they dread the awful amounts of practice time they think necessary to succeed on the test. We have refined an effective method that will take you only a fraction of the time.

There are a number of "obstacles" in your way to succeed. Among these are answering questions, finishing in time, and mastering test-taking strategies. All must be executed on the day of the test at peak performance, or your score will suffer. The test is a mental marathon that has a large impact on your future.

Just like a marathon runner, it is important to work your way up to the full challenge. So first you just worry about questions, and then time, and finally strategy:

Success Strategy

1. Find a good source for practice tests.
2. If you are willing to make a larger time investment, consider using more than one study guide- often the different approaches of multiple authors will help you "get" difficult concepts.
3. Take a practice test with no time constraints, with all study helps "open book." Take your time with questions and focus on applying strategies.
4. Take a practice test with time constraints, with all guides "open book."
5. Take a final practice test with no open material and time limits

If you have time to take more practice tests, just repeat step 5. By gradually exposing yourself to the full rigors of the test environment, you will condition your mind to the stress of test day and maximize your success.

Secret Key #4 - Prepare, Don't Procrastinate

Let me state an obvious fact: if you take the test three times, you will get three different scores. This is due to the way you feel on test day, the level of preparedness you have, and, despite the test writers' claims to the contrary, some tests WILL be easier for you than others.

Since your future depends so much on your score, you should maximize your chances of success. In order to maximize the likelihood of success, you've got to prepare in advance. This means taking practice tests and spending time learning the information and test taking strategies you will need to succeed.

Never take the test as a "practice" test, expecting that you can just take it again if you need to. Feel free to take sample tests on your own, but when you go to take the official test, be prepared, be focused, and do your best the first time!

Secret Key #5 - Test Yourself

Everyone knows that time is money. There is no need to spend too much of your time or too little of your time preparing for the test. You should only spend as much of your precious time preparing as is necessary for you to get the score you need.

Once you have taken a practice test under real conditions of time constraints, then you will know if you are ready for the test or not.

If you have scored extremely high the first time that you take the practice test, then there is not much point in spending countless hours studying. You are already there.

Benchmark your abilities by retaking practice tests and seeing how much you have improved. Once you score high enough to guarantee success, then you are ready.

If you have scored well below where you need, then knuckle down and begin studying in earnest. Check your improvement regularly through the use of practice tests under real conditions. Above all, don't worry, panic, or give up. The key is perseverance!

Then, when you go to take the test, remain confident and remember how well you did on the practice tests. If you can score high enough on a practice test, then you can do the same on the real thing.

General Strategies

The most important thing you can do is to ignore your fears and jump into the test immediately- do not be overwhelmed by any strange-sounding terms. You have to jump into the test like jumping into a pool- all at once is the easiest way.

Make Predictions

As you read and understand the question, try to guess what the answer will be. Remember that several of the answer choices are wrong, and once you begin reading them, your mind will immediately become cluttered with answer choices designed to throw you off. Your mind is typically the most focused immediately after you have read the question and digested its contents. If you can, try to predict what the correct answer will be. You may be surprised at what you can predict.

Quickly scan the choices and see if your prediction is in the listed answer choices. If it is, then you can be quite confident that you have the right answer. It still won't hurt to check the other answer choices, but most of the time, you've got it!

Answer the Question

It may seem obvious to only pick answer choices that answer the question, but the test writers can create some excellent answer choices that are wrong. Don't pick an answer just because it sounds right, or you believe it to be true. It MUST answer the question. Once you've made your selection, always go back and check it against the question and make sure that you didn't misread the question, and the answer choice does answer the question posed.

Benchmark

After you read the first answer choice, decide if you think it sounds correct or not. If it doesn't, move on to the next answer choice. If it does, mentally mark that answer choice. This doesn't mean that you've definitely selected it as your answer choice, it just means that it's the best you've seen thus far. Go ahead and read the next choice. If the next choice is worse than the one you've already selected, keep going to the next answer choice. If the next choice is better than the choice you've already selected, mentally mark the new answer choice as your best guess.

The first answer choice that you select becomes your standard. Every other answer choice must be benchmarked against that standard. That choice is correct until proven otherwise by another answer choice beating it out. Once you've decided that no other answer choice seems as good, do one final check to ensure that your answer choice answers the question posed.

Valid Information

Don't discount any of the information provided in the question. Every piece of information may be necessary to determine the correct answer. None of the information in the question is there to throw you off (while the answer choices will certainly have information to throw you off). If two seemingly unrelated topics are discussed, don't ignore either. You can be confident there is a relationship, or it wouldn't be included in the question, and you are probably going to have to determine what is that relationship to find the answer.

Avoid "Fact Traps"

Don't get distracted by a choice that is factually true. Your search is for the answer that answers the question. Stay focused and don't fall for an answer that is true but incorrect. Always go back to the question and make sure you're choosing an answer that actually answers the question and is not just a true statement. An answer can be factually correct, but it MUST answer the question asked. Additionally, two answers can both be seemingly correct, so be sure to read all of the answer choices, and make sure that you get the one that BEST answers the question.

Milk the Question

Some of the questions may throw you completely off. They might deal with a subject you have not been exposed to, or one that you haven't reviewed in years. While your lack of knowledge about the subject will be a hindrance, the question itself can give you many clues that will help you find the correct answer. Read the question carefully and look for clues. Watch particularly for adjectives and nouns describing difficult terms or words that you don't recognize. Regardless of if you completely understand a word or not, replacing it with a synonym either provided or one you more familiar with may help you to understand what the questions are asking. Rather than wracking your mind about specific detailed information concerning a difficult term or word, try to use mental substitutes that are easier to understand.

The Trap of Familiarity

Don't just choose a word because you recognize it. On difficult questions, you may not recognize a number of words in the answer choices. The test writers don't put "make-believe" words on the test; so don't think that just because you only recognize all the words in one answer choice means that answer choice must be correct. If you only recognize words in one answer choice, then focus on that one. Is it correct? Try your best to determine if it is correct. If it is, that is great, but if it doesn't, eliminate it. Each word and answer choice you eliminate increases your chances of getting the question correct, even if you then have to guess among the unfamiliar choices.

Eliminate Answers

Eliminate choices as soon as you realize they are wrong. But be careful! Make sure you consider all of the possible answer choices. Just because one appears right, doesn't mean that the next one won't be even better! The test writers will usually put more than one good answer choice for every question, so read all of them. Don't worry if you are stuck between two that seem right. By getting down to just two remaining possible choices, your odds are now 50/50. Rather than wasting too much time, play the odds. You are guessing, but guessing wisely, because you've been able to knock out some of the answer choices that you know are wrong. If you are eliminating choices and realize that the last answer choice you are left with is also obviously wrong, don't panic. Start over and consider each choice again. There may easily be something that you missed the first time and will realize on the second pass.

Tough Questions

If you are stumped on a problem or it appears too hard or too difficult, don't waste time. Move on! Remember though, if you can quickly check for obviously incorrect answer choices, your chances of guessing correctly are greatly improved. Before you completely give up, at least try to knock out a couple of possible answers. Eliminate what you can and then guess at the remaining answer choices before moving on.

Brainstorm

If you get stuck on a difficult question, spend a few seconds quickly brainstorming. Run through the complete list of possible answer choices. Look at each choice and ask yourself, "Could this answer the question satisfactorily?" Go through each answer choice and consider it independently of the other. By systematically going through all possibilities, you may find something that you would otherwise overlook. Remember that when you get stuck, it's important to try to keep moving.

Read Carefully

Understand the problem. Read the question and answer choices carefully. Don't miss the question because you misread the terms. You have plenty of time to read each question thoroughly and make sure you understand what is being asked. Yet a happy medium must be attained, so don't waste too much time. You must read carefully, but efficiently.

Face Value

When in doubt, use common sense. Always accept the situation in the problem at face value. Don't read too much into it. These problems will not require you to make huge leaps of logic. The test writers aren't trying to throw you off with a cheap trick. If you have to go beyond creativity and make a leap of logic in order to have an answer choice answer the question, then you should look at the other answer choices. Don't overcomplicate the problem by creating theoretical relationships or explanations that will warp time or space. These are normal problems rooted in reality. It's just that the applicable relationship or explanation may not be readily apparent and you have to figure things out. Use your common sense to interpret anything that isn't clear.

Prefixes

If you're having trouble with a word in the question or answer choices, try dissecting it. Take advantage of every clue that the word might include. Prefixes and suffixes can be a huge help. Usually they allow you to determine a basic meaning. Pre- means before, post- means after, pro - is positive, de- is negative. From these prefixes and suffixes, you can get an idea of the general meaning of the word and try to put it into context. Beware though of any traps. Just because con is the opposite of pro, doesn't necessarily mean congress is the opposite of progress!

Hedge Phrases

Watch out for critical "hedge" phrases, such as likely, may, can, will often, sometimes, often, almost, mostly, usually, generally, rarely, sometimes. Question writers insert these hedge phrases to cover every possibility. Often an answer choice will be wrong simply because it leaves no room for exception. Avoid answer choices that have definitive words like "exactly," and "always".

Switchback Words

Stay alert for "switchbacks". These are the words and phrases frequently used to alert you to shifts in thought. The most common switchback word is "but". Others include although, however, nevertheless, on the other hand, even though, while, in spite of, despite, regardless of.

New Information

Correct answer choices will rarely have completely new information included. Answer choices typically are straightforward reflections of the material asked about and will directly relate to the question. If a new piece of information is included in an answer choice that doesn't even seem to relate to the topic being asked about, then that answer choice is likely incorrect. All of the information needed to answer the question is usually provided for you, and so you should not have to make guesses that are unsupported or choose answer choices that require unknown information that cannot be reasoned on its own.

Time Management

On technical questions, don't get lost on the technical terms. Don't spend too much time on any one question. If you don't know what a term means, then since you don't have a dictionary, odds are you aren't going to get much further. You should immediately recognize terms as whether or not you know them. If you don't, work with the other clues that you have, the other answer choices and terms provided, but don't waste too much time trying to figure out a difficult term.

Contextual Clues

Look for contextual clues. An answer can be right but not correct. The contextual clues will help you find the answer that is most right and is correct. Understand the context in which a phrase or statement is made. This will help you make important distinctions.

Don't Panic

Panicking will not answer any questions for you. Therefore, it isn't helpful. When you first see the question, if your mind goes blank, take a deep breath. Force yourself to mechanically go through the steps of solving the problem and using the strategies you've learned.

Pace Yourself

Don't get clock fever. It's easy to be overwhelmed when you're looking at a page full of questions, your mind is full of random thoughts and feeling confused, and the clock is ticking down faster than you would like. Calm down and maintain the pace that you have set for yourself. As long as you are on track by monitoring your pace, you are guaranteed to have enough time for yourself. When you get to the last few minutes of the test, it may seem like you won't have enough time left, but if you only have as many questions as you should have left at that point, then you're right on track!

Answer Selection

The best way to pick an answer choice is to eliminate all of those that are wrong, until only one is left and confirm that is the correct answer. Sometimes though, an answer choice may immediately look right. Be careful! Take a second to make sure that the other choices are not equally obvious. Don't make a hasty mistake. There are only two times that you should stop before checking other answers. First is when you are positive that the answer choice you have selected is correct. Second is when time is almost out and you have to make a quick guess!

Check Your Work

Since you will probably not know every term listed and the answer to every question, it is important that you get credit for the ones that you do know. Don't miss any questions through careless mistakes. If at all possible, try to take a second to look back over your answer selection and make sure you've selected the correct answer choice and haven't made a costly careless mistake (such as marking an answer choice that you didn't mean to mark). This quick double check should more than pay for itself in caught mistakes for the time it costs.

Beware of Directly Quoted Answers

Sometimes an answer choice will repeat word for word a portion of the question or reference section. However, beware of such exact duplication – it may be a trap! More than likely, the correct choice will paraphrase or summarize a point, rather than being exactly the same wording.

Slang

Scientific sounding answers are better than slang ones. An answer choice that begins "To compare the outcomes..." is much more likely to be correct than one that begins "Because some people insisted..."

Extreme Statements

Avoid wild answers that throw out highly controversial ideas that are proclaimed as established fact. An answer choice that states the "process should be used in certain situations, if..." is much more likely to be correct than one that states the "process should be discontinued completely." The first is a calm rational statement and doesn't even make a definitive, uncompromising stance, using a hedge word "if" to provide wiggle room, whereas the second choice is a radical idea and far more extreme.

Answer Choice Families

When you have two or more answer choices that are direct opposites or parallels, one of them is usually the correct answer. For instance, if one answer choice states "x increases" and another answer choice states "x decreases" or "y increases," then those two or three answer choices are very similar in construction and fall into the same family of answer choices. A family of answer choices is when two or three answer choices are very similar in construction, and yet often have a directly opposite meaning.   Usually the correct answer choice will be in that family of answer choices. The "odd man out" or answer choice that doesn't seem to fit the parallel construction of the other answer choices is more likely to be incorrect.

Special Report: How to Overcome Test Anxiety

The very nature of tests caters to some level of anxiety, nervousness or tension, just as we feel for any important event that occurs in our lives. A little bit of anxiety or nervousness can be a good thing. It helps us with motivation, and makes achievement just that much sweeter. However, too much anxiety can be a problem; especially if it hinders our ability to function and perform.

"Test anxiety," is the term that refers to the emotional reactions that some test-takers experience when faced with a test or exam. Having a fear of testing and exams is based upon a rational fear, since the test-taker's performance can shape the course of an academic career. Nevertheless, experiencing excessive fear of examinations will only interfere with the test-takers ability to perform, and his/her chances to be successful.

There are a large variety of causes that can contribute to the development and sensation of test anxiety. These include, but are not limited to lack of performance and worrying about issues surrounding the test.

Lack of Preparation

Lack of preparation can be identified by the following behaviors or situations:

Not scheduling enough time to study, and therefore cramming the night before the test or exam
Managing time poorly, to create the sensation that there is not enough time to do everything

Failing to organize the text information in advance, so that the study material consists of the entire text and not simply the pertinent information

Poor overall studying habits

Worrying, on the other hand, can be related to both the test taker, or many other factors around him/her that will be affected by the results of the test. These include worrying about:

Previous performances on similar exams, or exams in general

How friends and other students are achieving

The negative consequences that will result from a poor grade or failure

There are three primary elements to test anxiety. Physical components, which involve the same typical bodily reactions as those to acute anxiety (to be discussed below). Emotional factors have to do with fear or panic. Mental or cognitive issues concerning attention spans and memory abilities.

Physical Signals

There are many different symptoms of test anxiety, and these are not limited to mental and emotional strain. Frequently there are a range of physical signals that will let a test taker know that he/she is suffering from test anxiety. These bodily changes can include the following:

Perspiring

Sweaty palms

Wet, trembling hands

Nausea

Dry mouth

A knot in the stomach

Headache

Faintness

Muscle tension

Aching shoulders, back and neck

Rapid heart beat

Feeling too hot/cold

To recognize the sensation of test anxiety, a test-taker should monitor him/herself for the following sensations:

The physical distress symptoms as listed above

Emotional sensitivity, expressing emotional feelings such as the need to cry or laugh too much, or a sensation of anger or helplessness

A decreased ability to think, causing the test-taker to blank out or have racing thoughts that are hard to organize or control.

Though most students will feel some level of anxiety when faced with a test or exam, the majority can cope with that anxiety and maintain it at a manageable level. However, those who cannot are faced with a very real and very serious condition, which can and should be controlled for the immeasurable benefit of this sufferer.

Naturally, these sensations lead to negative results for the testing experience. The most common effects of test anxiety have to do with nervousness and mental blocking.

Nervousness

Nervousness can appear in several different levels:

The test-taker's difficulty, or even inability to read and understand the questions on the test

The difficulty or inability to organize thoughts to a coherent form

The difficulty or inability to recall key words and concepts relating to the testing questions (especially essays)

The receipt of poor grades on a test, though the test material was well known by the test taker

Conversely, a person may also experience mental blocking, which involves:

Blanking out on test questions

Only remembering the correct answers to the questions when the test has already finished.

Fortunately for test anxiety sufferers, beating these feelings, to a large degree, has to do with proper preparation. When a test taker has a feeling of preparedness, then anxiety will be dramatically lessened.

The first step to resolving anxiety issues is to distinguish which of the two types of anxiety are being suffered. If the anxiety is a direct result of a lack of preparation, this should be considered a normal reaction, and the anxiety level (as opposed to the test results) shouldn't be anything to worry about. However, if, when adequately prepared, the test-taker still panics, blanks out, or seems to overreact, this is not a fully rational reaction. While this can be considered normal too, there are many ways to combat and overcome these effects.

Remember that anxiety cannot be entirely eliminated, however, there are ways to minimize it, to make the anxiety easier to manage. Preparation is one of the best ways to minimize test anxiety. Therefore the following techniques are wise in order to best fight off any anxiety that may want to build.

To begin with, try to avoid cramming before a test, whenever it is possible. By trying to memorize an entire term's worth of information in one day, you'll be shocking your system, and not giving yourself a very good chance to absorb the information. This is an easy path to anxiety, so for those who suffer from test anxiety, cramming should not even be considered an option.

Instead of cramming, work throughout the semester to combine all of the material which is presented throughout the semester, and work on it gradually as the course goes by, making sure to master the main concepts first, leaving minor details for a week or so before the test.

To study for the upcoming exam, be sure to pose questions that may be on the examination, to gauge the ability to answer them by integrating the ideas from your texts, notes and lectures, as well as any supplementary readings.

If it is truly impossible to cover all of the information that was covered in that particular term, concentrate on the most important portions, that can be covered very well. Learn these concepts as best as possible, so that when the test comes, a goal can be made to use these concepts as presentations of your knowledge.

In addition to study habits, changes in attitude are critical to beating a struggle with test anxiety. In fact, an improvement of the perspective over the entire test-taking experience can actually help a test taker to enjoy studying and therefore improve the overall experience. Be certain not to overemphasize the significance of the grade - know that the result of the test is neither a reflection of self worth, nor is it a measure of intelligence; one grade will not predict a person's future success.

To improve an overall testing outlook, the following steps should be tried:

Keeping in mind that the most reasonable expectation for taking a test is to expect to try to demonstrate as much of what you know as you possibly can. Reminding ourselves that a test is only one test; this is not the only one, and there will be others.

The thought of thinking of oneself in an irrational, all-or-nothing term should be avoided at all costs.

A reward should be designated for after the test, so there's something to look forward to. Whether it be going to a movie, going out to eat, or simply visiting friends, schedule it in advance, and do it no matter what result is expected on the exam.

Test-takers should also keep in mind that the basics are some of the most important things, even beyond anti-anxiety techniques and studying. Never neglect the basic social, emotional and biological needs, in order to try to absorb information. In order to best achieve, these three factors must be held as just as important as the studying itself.

Study Steps

Remember the following important steps for studying:

Maintain healthy nutrition and exercise habits. Continue both your recreational activities and social pass times. These both contribute to your physical and emotional well being.

Be certain to get a good amount of sleep, especially the night before the test, because when you're overtired you are not able to perform to the best of your best ability.

Keep the studying pace to a moderate level by taking breaks when they are needed, and varying the work whenever possible, to keep the mind fresh instead of getting bored.

When enough studying has been done that all the material that can be learned has been learned, and the test taker is prepared for the test, stop studying and do something relaxing such as listening to music, watching a movie, or taking a warm bubble bath.

There are also many other techniques to minimize the uneasiness or apprehension that is experienced along with test anxiety before, during, or even after the examination. In fact, there are a great deal of things that can be done to stop anxiety from interfering with lifestyle and performance. Again, remember that anxiety will not be eliminated entirely, and it shouldn't be. Otherwise that "up" feeling for exams would not exist, and most of us depend on that sensation to perform better than usual. However, this anxiety has to be at a level that is manageable.

Of course, as we have just discussed, being prepared for the exam is half the battle right away. Attending all classes, finding out what knowledge will be expected on the exam, and knowing the exam schedules are easy steps to lowering anxiety. Keeping up with work will remove the need to cram, and efficient study habits will eliminate wasted time. Studying should be done in an ideal location for concentration, so that it is simple to become interested in the material and give it complete attention. A method such as SQ3R (Survey, Question, Read, Recite, Review) is a wonderful key to follow to make sure that the study habits are as effective as possible, especially in the case of learning from a textbook. Flashcards are great techniques for memorization. Learning to take good notes will mean that notes will be full of useful information, so that less sifting will need to be done to seek out what is pertinent for studying. Reviewing notes after class and then again on occasion will keep the information fresh in the mind. From notes that have been taken summary sheets and outlines can be made for simpler reviewing.

A study group can also be a very motivational and helpful place to study, as there will be a sharing of ideas, all of the minds can work together, to make sure that everyone understands, and the studying will be made more interesting because it will be a social occasion.

Basically, though, as long as the test-taker remains organized and self confident, with efficient study habits, less time will need to be spent studying, and higher grades will be achieved.

To become self confident, there are many useful steps. The first of these is "self talk." It has been shown through extensive research, that self-talk for students who suffer from test anxiety, should be well monitored, in order to make sure that it contributes to self confidence as opposed to sinking the student. Frequently the self talk of test-anxious students is negative or self-defeating, thinking that everyone else is smarter and faster, that they always mess up, and that if they don't do well, they'll fail the entire course. It is important to decreasing anxiety that awareness is made of self talk. Try writing any negative self thoughts and then disputing them with a positive statement instead. Begin self-encouragement as though it was a friend speaking. Repeat positive statements to help reprogram the mind to believing in successes instead of failures.

Helpful Techniques

Other extremely helpful techniques include:

Self-visualization of doing well and reaching goals

While aiming for an "A" level of understanding, don't try to "overprotect" by setting your expectations lower. This will only convince the mind to stop studying in order to meet the lower expectations.

Don't make comparisons with the results or habits of other students. These are individual factors, and different things work for different people, causing different results.

Strive to become an expert in learning what works well, and what can be done in order to improve. Consider collecting this data in a journal.

Create rewards for after studying instead of doing things before studying that will only turn into avoidance behaviors.

Make a practice of relaxing - by using methods such as progressive relaxation, self-hypnosis, guided imagery, etc - in order to make relaxation an automatic sensation.

Work on creating a state of relaxed concentration so that concentrating will take on the focus of the mind, so that none will be wasted on worrying.

Take good care of the physical self by eating well and getting enough sleep.

Plan in time for exercise and stick to this plan.

Beyond these techniques, there are other methods to be used before, during and after the test that will help the test-taker perform well in addition to overcoming anxiety.

Before the exam comes the academic preparation. This involves establishing a study schedule and beginning at least one week before the actual date of the test. By doing this, the anxiety of not having enough time to study for the test will be automatically eliminated. Moreover, this will make the studying a much more effective experience, ensuring that the learning will be an easier process. This relieves much undue pressure on the test-taker.

Summary sheets, note cards, and flash cards with the main concepts and examples of these main concepts should be prepared in advance of the actual studying time. A topic should never be eliminated from this process. By omitting a topic because it isn't expected to be on the test is only setting up the test-taker for anxiety should it actually appear on the exam. Utilize the course syllabus for laying out the topics that should be studied. Carefully go over the notes that were made in class, paying special attention to any of the issues that the professor took special care to emphasize while lecturing in class. In the textbooks, use the chapter review, or if possible, the chapter tests, to begin your review.

It may even be possible to ask the instructor what information will be covered on the exam, or what the format of the exam will be (for example, multiple choice, essay, free form, true-false). Additionally, see if it is possible to find out how many questions will be on the test. If a review sheet or sample test has been offered by the professor, make good use of it, above anything else, for the preparation for the test. Another great resource for getting to know the examination is reviewing tests from previous semesters. Use these tests to review, and aim to achieve a 100% score on each of the possible topics. With a few exceptions, the goal that you set for yourself is the highest one that you will reach.

Take all of the questions that were assigned as homework, and rework them to any other possible course material. The more problems reworked, the more skill and confidence will form as a result. When forming the solution to a problem, write out each of the steps. Don't simply do head work. By doing as many steps on paper as possible, much clarification and therefore confidence will be formed. Do this with as many homework problems as possible, before checking the answers. By checking the answer after each problem, a reinforcement will exist, that will not be on the exam. Study situations should be as exam-like as possible, to prime the test-taker's system for the experience. By waiting to check the answers at the end, a psychological advantage will be formed, to decrease the stress factor.

Another fantastic reason for not cramming is the avoidance of confusion in concepts, especially when it comes to mathematics. 8-10 hours of study will become one hundred percent more effective if it is spread out over a week or at least several days, instead of doing it all in one sitting. Recognize that the human brain requires time in order to assimilate new material, so frequent breaks and a span of study time over several days will be much more beneficial.

Additionally, don't study right up until the point of the exam. Studying should stop a minimum of one hour before the exam begins. This allows the brain to rest and put things in their proper order. This will also provide the time to become as relaxed as possible when going into the examination room. The test-taker will also have time to eat well and eat sensibly. Know that the brain needs food as much as the rest of the body. With enough food and enough sleep, as well as a relaxed attitude, the body and the mind are primed for success.

Avoid any anxious classmates who are talking about the exam. These students only spread anxiety, and are not worth sharing the anxious sentimentalities.

Before the test also involves creating a positive attitude, so mental preparation should also be a point of concentration. There are many keys to creating a positive attitude. Should fears become rushing in, make a visualization of taking the exam, doing well, and seeing an A written on the paper. Write out a list of affirmations that will bring a feeling of confidence, such as "I am doing well in my English class," "I studied well and know my material," "I enjoy this class." Even if the affirmations aren't believed at first, it sends a positive message to the subconscious which will result in an alteration of the overall belief system, which is the system that creates reality.

If a sensation of panic begins, work with the fear and imagine the very worst! Work through the entire scenario of not passing the test, failing the entire course, and dropping out of school, followed by not getting a job, and pushing a shopping cart through the dark alley where you'll live. This will place things into perspective! Then, practice deep breathing and create a visualization of the opposite situation - achieving an "A" on the exam, passing the entire course, receiving the degree at a graduation ceremony.

On the day of the test, there are many things to be done to ensure the best results, as well as the most calm outlook. The following stages are suggested in order to maximize test-taking potential:

Begin the examination day with a moderate breakfast, and avoid any coffee or beverages with caffeine if the test taker is prone to jitters. Even people who are used to managing caffeine can feel jittery or light-headed when it is taken on a test day.

Attempt to do something that is relaxing before the examination begins. As last minute cramming clouds the mastering of overall concepts, it is better to use this time to create a calming outlook.

Be certain to arrive at the test location well in advance, in order to provide time to select a location that is away from doors, windows and other distractions, as well as giving enough time to relax before the test begins.

Keep away from anxiety generating classmates who will upset the sensation of stability and relaxation that is being attempted before the exam.

Should the waiting period before the exam begins cause anxiety, create a self-distraction by reading a light magazine or something else that is relaxing and simple.

During the exam itself, read the entire exam from beginning to end, and find out how much time should be allotted to each individual problem. Once writing the exam, should more time be taken for a problem, it should be abandoned, in order to begin another problem. If there is time at the end, the unfinished problem can always be returned to and completed.

Read the instructions very carefully - twice - so that unpleasant surprises won't follow during or after the exam has ended.

When writing the exam, pretend that the situation is actually simply the completion of homework within a library, or at home. This will assist in forming a relaxed atmosphere, and will allow the brain extra focus for the complex thinking function.

Begin the exam with all of the questions with which the most confidence is felt. This will build the confidence level regarding the entire exam and will begin a quality momentum. This will also create encouragement for trying the problems where uncertainty resides.

Going with the "gut instinct" is always the way to go when solving a problem. Second guessing should be avoided at all costs. Have confidence in the ability to do well.

For essay questions, create an outline in advance that will keep the mind organized and make certain that all of the points are remembered. For multiple choice, read every answer, even if the correct one has been spotted - a better one may exist.

Continue at a pace that is reasonable and not rushed, in order to be able to work carefully. Provide enough time to go over the answers at the end, to check for small errors that can be corrected.

Should a feeling of panic begin, breathe deeply, and think of the feeling of the body releasing sand through its pores. Visualize a calm, peaceful place, and include all of the sights, sounds and sensations of this image. Continue the deep breathing, and take a few minutes to continue this with closed eyes. When all is well again, return to the test.

If a "blanking" occurs for a certain question, skip it and move on to the next question. There will be time to return to the other question later. Get everything done that can be done, first, to guarantee all the grades that can be compiled, and to build all of the confidence possible. Then return to the weaker questions to build the marks from there.

Remember, one's own reality can be created, so as long as the belief is there, success will follow. And remember: anxiety can happen later, right now, there's an exam to be written!

After the examination is complete, whether there is a feeling for a good grade or a bad grade, don't dwell on the exam, and be certain to follow through on the reward that was promised…and enjoy it! Don't dwell on any mistakes that have been made, as there is nothing that can be done at this point anyway.

Additionally, don't begin to study for the next test right away. Do something relaxing for a while, and let the mind relax and prepare itself to begin absorbing information again.

From the results of the exam - both the grade and the entire experience, be certain to learn from what has gone on. Perfect studying habits and work some more on confidence in order to make the next examination experience even better than the last one.

Learn to avoid places where openings occurred for laziness, procrastination and day dreaming.

Use the time between this exam and the next one to better learn to relax, even learning to relax on cue, so that any anxiety can be controlled during the next exam. Learn how to relax the body. Slouch in your chair if that helps. Tighten and then relax all of the different muscle groups, one group at a time, beginning with the feet and then working all the way up to the neck and face. This will ultimately relax the muscles more than they were to begin with. Learn how to breathe deeply and comfortably, and focus on this breathing going in and out as a relaxing thought. With every exhale, repeat the word "relax."

As common as test anxiety is, it is very possible to overcome it. Make yourself one of the test-takers who overcome this frustrating hindrance.

Special Report: Additional Bonus Material

Due to our efforts to try to keep this book to a manageable length, we've created a link that will give you access to all of your additional bonus material.

Please visit http://www.mometrix.com/bonus948/nursingadmin to access the information.